Heart Health

Heart Health

A Guide to the Tests and Treatments You Really Need

J Shah, MD

ROWMAN & LITTLEFIELD
Lanham • Boulder • New York • London

Published by Rowman & Littlefield
An imprint of The Rowman & Littlefield Publishing Group, Inc.
4501 Forbes Boulevard, Suite 200, Lanham, Maryland 20706
www.rowman.com

6 Tinworth Street, London SE11 5AL, United Kingdom

British Library Cataloguing in Publication Information Available

Library of Congress Cataloging-in-Publication Data

Names: Shah, J, author.
Title: Heart health : A guide to the tests and treatments you really need / J Shah, MD.
Description: London ; New York : Rowman & Littlefield Publishers, 2019. | Includes
    bibliographical references and index.
Identifiers: LCCN 2019001929| ISBN 9781538126691 (cloth : alk. paper) | ISBN
    9781538126707 (electronic)
Subjects: LCSH: Heart—Examination. | Heart—Diseases—Treatment.
Classification: LCC RC683 .S52 2019 | DDC 616.1/2075—dc23 LC record
    available at https://lccn.loc.gov/2019001929

To my mother,
who gave me the thirst for knowledge

To my father,
who taught me the discipline to acquire it

Contents

List of Figures

List of Tables

Acknowledgments

This book, as all endeavors of an individual, is a team effort. My team included family and friends who have made me the person I have become and the doctor I yearn to be day after day.

My brother Ketan has been by my side through the thick and thin of my struggles of being a renegade doctor. He has supported me in good times and bad, in my exhilarations and frustrations, success and failures, without judging, prodding, or blaming but always encouraging and cheering. He has been instrumental in reviewing some of the drafts before the drafts, ideas before they were completed in my mind, and bearing the repetition of my thoughts about the contents of this book. He reviewed every chapter with the detail that only a brother would, despite battling several competing priorities.

My girlfriend Rebecca, who I ignored for many months while I spent time working on the book, reviewed every chapter, making suggestions in her gentle way.

My dear nephews and nieces: Nisarg for taking the lead on reviewing the book and making awesome suggestions; his enthusiasm for the hooks in the stories was encouraging; Zeel and Veeksha for encouraging me to be a better writer and reviewing the book.

Nilesh Chatterjee, who initiated me to write and helped me all along; he patiently edited my nonsensical writing and make it worth a read. Sreeram Sivaramakrisnan, editing some of my work and pointing me to other works related to this subject.

My aunt Deepika for initiating the passion of reading and encouraging me throughout the process of my book.

Lynne, who reviewed every chapter in detail and lived the emotions of the patients in every chapter. Without Lynne this book would be altogether insipid.

Lauren Whalen who made the characters and stories come alive in every chapter and made them larger than life. Lauren made me a better writer by reviewing and editing early drafts in every minor detail possible.

KiranFua who believed that I am capable of writing and have worthwhile thoughts to be put on paper to be read by others.

Dr. H. Gilbert Welch who encouraged me to start the book and gave several suggestions that became the guiding principles throughout my writing process.

Introduction

Why Do I Need This Book?

> The doctor of the future will give no medicine, but will interest his patient
> in the care of the human frame, in diet and in the cause and prevention
> of disease.
>
> —Thomas Edison[1]

Medical science has made immense progress over the years, prolonging the lives of millions and improving the lives of millions more. However, navigating the health-care system is complicated and frightening for most people. This task becomes all the more challenging when one considers the physical limitations and anxiety caused by illness, confusion over medical jargon, the pressure of making the right decision, and the cost of medication and procedures. All these factors leave patients feeling overwhelmed and helpless, who land up deferring to physicians and the system to make a choice for them.

When it comes to heart-related issues, the problem is further intensified. All around us, there are billboards, stories, television programs, and newspaper articles related to heart disease. The media bombards us with fear of the "epidemic" of heart disease and the havoc it can wreak on one's life. This leaves patients believing that when it comes to heart-related issues one has to be immensely cautious. They believe that the heart and all its components have to work with 100 percent perfection, 100 percent of the time, and anything less is a sign of impending doom. The accepted course of action, therefore, is to seek care immediately and follow through on all and every available treatment to avoid near-certain death. This is a myth that has been promoted by laypeople and professionals alike.

The truth, however, is more nuanced.

A large majority of heart diseases are no different than other chronic diseases like diabetes or arthritis insofar as the required urgency of treatment is concerned. Consider this: If all three arteries of your heart are 70 to 80 percent blocked, your average life expectancy when these are treated with medicine alone is eight years, and bypass surgery can increase this life expectancy by around six months.[2] So, though bypass surgery is helpful and necessary in many cases, it is not saving you from *impending* death, as the system would have you believe. All too often, patients are rushed into bypass surgeries as a case of dire emergency even though there is plenty of time to get a second opinion, get on the right medicine, and consider bypass surgery over the course of a few weeks.

Consider another example of congestive heart failure. Even the very mention of congestive heart failure evokes dramatic anxiety among patients as if it were a death sentence. In reality, congestive heart failure is a spectrum of diseases, with the severity level ranging from mild—that is, where the patient is able to perform all activities—to moderate—that is, where the patient suffers shortness of breath when performing routine day-to-day activities—and all the way to the more advanced stages—that is, where the patient might become short of breath from just sitting up in bed. As one can imagine, the long-term outlook between these groups of patients with congestive heart failure varies.

All in all, different severity of heart diseases have different impact on quality of life and need different level of urgency and attention. The majority of heart conditions neither pose immediate peril to life nor require emergency tests and treatments but patients feel crippled when given the diagnosis of heart disease and automatically assume they are at death's door.

This false belief has been widely propagated by aggressive marketing from invested parties using multiple media outlets.

The narrative that naturally follows this myth—that heart disease means sure death—is that doctors can fix this problem using surgeries and modern devices and save your life. Though in a minority of emergency circumstances this may be true, the majority of diseases can be prevented with diet, exercise, weight control, blood sugar control, and blood pressure control.[3] Furthermore, most heart diseases can be treated with medication, though in some cases procedures, surgeries, and devices may also be required to treat the disease. The procedures, surgeries, and devices that were invented in the twentieth century have saved the lives of many *when used under the right conditions*. However, these "advanced" technological procedures have taken on the central role in today's management of heart disease. While they have been of use in treating the types of diseases they were invented for, the reckless use of these technologies can and does wreak havoc on the lives of many patients who may not need them. These procedures add little or negligible value to a patient's longevity or quality of life when used imprudently.

Studies have shown that in regions of the United States with more hospital beds per capita, patients are more likely to be admitted to the hospital. In regions where there are more intensive care–unit beds, more patients will be cared for there in the ICU. More specialist availability means more patients see those specialists. And the more CT scanners that are available means more orders for CT scans.[4] It's quite the case of supply creating its own demand!

Similarly, in regions where there are more cardiologists and cardiac surgeons, there are more procedures, more surgeries, and more expenses. And yet the patients who receive this extra "care" neither live longer nor enjoy improved quality of life despite these extra procedures and surgeries. In fact, the care they receive appears to be worse. Historically, these patients are less satisfied with their care, do not live longer, and incur much higher medical expenses.[5]

So, why does this happen, and what can be done about it?

There are several reasons why patients receive procedures, surgeries, and devices that may or may not benefit them.

First, these procedures, surgeries, and devices bring lots more money to hospitals and doctors compared to clinic visits, informative conversation, and the use of medicine. This lopsided incentive ensures that doctors are inclined to offer procedures as the best option while overlooking the potential use of equally effective but less-invasive and cheaper alternative.[6] We have left the policing of the doctors to the free market. However, as William Sage, doctor, lawyer, and professor of Health Law at the University of Texas, says "Medicine is a business. It won't police itself. People had a lot of faith in the American medical profession—that they would act differently than other businesses— but they were wrong."[7]

The second reason so many patients receive unnecessary procedures, surgeries, and devices stems from the myth that any heart condition is a sign of impending death, which has primed patients and family members to accept all suggested tests and surgeries. There is a pervasive belief that more testing and treatment is better, so clinicians, patients, and family members alike have a bias in favor of performing tests and procedures rather than opting for observation and medication and *then*, finally, if needed, moving to consider procedures and surgeries.[8] As a result, many patients undergo cardiac procedures even when other competing illnesses are already gnawing away at their survival. In cases where patients with advanced age and dementia undergo complex valve surgeries, for example, the patient is unlikely to notice any increase in lifespan. It will be a matter of choosing one cause of death—here dementia—over another—here cardiac death.

The third reason procedures, surgeries, and devices are overused to treat cardiac patients is because among both physicians and patients there is a technological imperative—the idea that new technologies are better and must be adopted for the benefit of all.[9] On an individual level, patients believe that newer technology is better and improves longevity and quality of life much more than medicine can. While this may be true in a small minority of cases, the majority of the time, newer technology makes marginal improvement if any and potentially comes at a higher cost and risk of complications.[10]

Given the present climate surrounding medical care, the goal of this book is to provide present and potential patients and their family members a tool to navigate the maze of cardiac procedures. Having spent twenty years training and practicing medicine at premier institutes across several countries, I believe that if the reckless use of procedure, overdiagnosis, and overtreatment is eliminated, American medicine can deliver its very best care to millions. This book is neither a policy guide nor a primer on healthcare economics but rather is focused on individual patients and their heart health. It aims to provide an understanding of various procedures, surgeries, and devices involved in heart care, put them into perspective, and discuss the good, the bad, and the ugly of such ubiquitous technologies.

The book is divided into several chapters, each focusing on a cardiac test or procedure. Each offers a fictional patient story, drawn from a composite of my experiences with patients, followed by a brief history of the "invention" of the procedure. In the latter half of each chapter, the patient story continues, highlighting the devolution of the procedure in the American healthcare system. Finally, the appendix of each chapter offers the reader a deeper understanding of the procedure itself, what it entails, and more importantly the right questions to consider prior to consenting to the procedure.

By the end of the book, I hope you take away the following key lessons on how to navigate the world of heart health:

- A healthy diet, exercise, weight control, blood sugar control, and blood pressure control ("home-care system") is much more impactful in preventing and managing heart disease than are procedures or surgeries (the health-care system).
- When offered tests or procedures ask questions about the *impact* of the procedure: Will it prolong your life? Will it improve the quality of your life?

- When offered tests and procedures ask questions about the *specific risks and complications* involved.
- Carefully compare the risks of the procedures and surgeries against their benefits. If the benefits outweigh the risks, the procedure is justified.
- Do not rush or allow yourself to be rushed into procedures or surgeries. In the majority of cases, there is ample time to weigh the risks and benefits, as well as seek a second opinion before opting for procedures. Except in an emergency situation where you have been rushed to the emergency room with chest pain and shortness of breath, etc., a second opinion is always a good idea.
- Visit reputable websites for healthcare information with no commercial bias.

If this book makes you a more-informed consumer of cardiac care by guiding you on the role of observation, medicine, procedures, and surgeries, it will have served its purpose. If this book causes you to refrain from rushing into unnecessary cardiac procedures and instead guides you to seek a second opinion, it will have served its purpose. And most importantly, if this book convinces you to improve your home-care system—your diet, exercise, weight control, blood sugar control, and blood pressure control—before turning to the health-care system, it will have served its purpose.

I hope you use this book to get the best cardiac care in the world.

—J. Shah, MD

> The inexperienced & presumptuous band of medical tyros let loose upon the world, destroys more of human life in one year, than all the Robinhoods, Cartouches, & Macheaths do in a century. It is in this part of medicine that I wish to see a reform, an abandonment of hypothesis for sober facts, the first degree of value set on clinical observation, and the lowest on visionary theories.
>
> —Thomas Jefferson[11]

> The best doctor gives the least medicine.
>
> —Benjamin Franklin[12]

1

Stress Test: What's Good for the Goose Good for the Gander?

There is no one-size-fits-all narrative; everyone's path winds in different ways.

—Sarah McBride[1]

STRESS TEST,
AKA EXERCISE STRESS TEST,
TREADMILL TEST

Loneliness Breeds Unexpected Friendships

They were both transplants to Florida, having moved there after spending a lifetime in the Northeast. Their commonality ended there. Susan was a retired schoolteacher from Vermont, whereas Barbara had been a senior manager in New Jersey. Susan was a simple, laid-back, but well-read woman who had never married and didn't have a large family, whereas Barbara was a fashionable go-getter, a jet-setter who had traveled the world, was twice divorced, and belonged to a large, close-knit family. Susan enjoyed yoga and meditation and loved the smell of a new book, while Barbara enjoyed great wine, spent a lot of time on the Internet, and connected with her friends late into the night.

They had both moved into a new subdivision outside of Metro Orlando, an area teeming with lakes and walking paths. Three-fourths of the housing units were still empty, so their neighborhood of eighty houses felt intimate. Families often came together for backyard gatherings, shooting hoops, and playing card games.

The two women had met during one of the summer barbeques. Their differences melted away in the lonely subdivision, and they became friends. On Susan's seventy-first birthday, Barbara had expressed anxiety about her own impending seventieth birthday and the importance of making health a priority. The two resolved to start walking together regularly.

What had started on a whim quickly became a cherished ritual for both of them. Over the course of their regular walking routine, they became closer, discovering similar interests in book genres, hobbies, and life lessons. Soon, they became fast friends, loyal confidants, and treasured companions.

What Are Good Friends For?

During their more recent walks, Barbara had started noticing that their pace had slowed down and that they were taking much longer to get through their usual circuit. On more than a few occasions lately Susan had asked to do a shorter circuit, though she had assured a surprised Barbara that it was for no particular reason. Barbara had also noted that Susan stopped to rest more often, which seemed very unusual. Susan had revealed in the past that she had high blood pressure but other than that, no medical conditions. After about fifteen days of this stop-and-go walking, during yet another rest stop, Barbara could no longer ignore it.

"How are you feeling, Susan?"

"Okay—just catching my breath." Susan bent over, avoiding Barbara's concerned gaze.

"I want to make sure that you're okay. You've had to stop to catch a breath too frequently of late, and you haven't been at your usual marching speed for a while," Barbara worried aloud.

"It's the cold I caught around Christmas," Susan explained with a dismissive wave of her hand.

"It is taking a long time to clear out. The Fourth of July is around the corner," Barbara pressed.

"Yes, my doctor said it takes a while." Susan straightened, closing the conversation before Barbara could reply, and they continued walking.

When they had reached the end of the walk and started driving home, Susan found her words again. "My doctor told me back in February that sometimes it takes a while to get over a cold, but you're right. It has been four months since then, and I still can't seem to get my breath back. I wonder if I should check with her."

Barbara patted her hand. "There's no harm in getting checked out. If you want me to go with you, let me know. I am happy to accompany you to the doctor's office."

Barbara had always believed that four ears are better than two at the doctor's office and was keen to help her friend.

"Let me see when they can fit me in, and I'll let you know." Susan resolved to call the doctor's office that afternoon.

At the Doctor's Office

On the day of the appointment, Susan and Barbara left early to beat the traffic. At the doctor's office, once they had taken care of the paperwork, the assistant took them back to the patient room. Dr. Wilson entered. She was surprised to see Susan sooner than her scheduled six-month appointment and asked with concern what the problem was.

"My breathing has not improved since the cold I caught in December," Susan explained.

Dr. Wilson took Susan through a series of questions about fever, chills, chest pain, coughs, leg swelling, and other symptoms. She then questioned her about blood pressure control and whether Susan was regular with her meds. Finally, she performed an examination.

"Your lungs are clear, your heart sounds good, and I am not finding anything wrong," she summarized.

"Then why do I get short-winded? This is very unusual." Susan was audibly disappointed; she had been hoping that the doctor would just give her some medicine to fix it.

"I agree. I think we need to check it out with a few tests. Shortness of breath can be due to heart, lung, or blood count–related problems, so I suggest that we send out some blood work, check a chest X-ray, and get a stress test. They will give us some answers." She kept her eyes down, scribbling notes on Susan's chart.

"You think this could be my heart?" asked Susan, surprised. "I have no chest pain at all, my blood pressure is under good control, and I take my meds regularly."

"Shortness of breath can definitely be caused by a heart problem, such as blockages in the heart arteries or weakness in pumping. It's not unusual to have heart problems at your age, especially with your high blood pressure and family history of heart conditions. Yes, we should definitely check your heart for the cause of your shortness of breath, since it is a common connection. The stress test is an indirect way of finding out if there are blockages in the heart arteries. If these tests are normal we can look into other tests to look for something more rare that might be causing it," Dr. Wilson clarified.

She was a strong believer in open communication and invariably found time to explain what was needed and why.

It Can't Be My Heart

"But I've never had any heart issues! I eat a healthy diet, Barbara and I walk three miles every day, and I have never smoked in my entire life. Didn't you mention that my cholesterol was good just last year?" Susan was insistent; it would be unfair for her to have heart disease after how careful she had been with her health!

Dr. Wilson paused for a moment, then put her hand on Susan's, and smiled. "I know it can be stressful to think that you may have a heart problem." She noticed that Susan's tense muscles relaxed a little at her words, and continued. "You are doing everything you can to avoid heart problems, I know. However, given the risk factors of age, your history of high blood pressure, and the family history of heart disease, it's still a possibility." She made sure to stress the last word while looking Susan in the eye. "I hope this is not the case, and the stress test is normal, but I still think it's prudent to check."

"What do they do in a stress test?" Barbara chimed in. She knew Susan was too distraught to ask anything else.

"They attach EKG wires to you and inject a radioactive dye through your IV. The dye goes through the heart arteries to the heart muscles that receive the blood supply, which will brighten up when they take pictures. Then they have you walk-run on a treadmill, and after exercise they inject the dye again and once again take pictures. The before and after exercise pictures are then compared. If the rest picture is good but the exercise picture is defective, it will tell us that a heart muscle is not receiving adequate blood supply when you exercise. This indicates that there are blockages in the arteries. On the other hand, if the rest and exercise pictures both look good, you don't have blockages in the heart arteries, and we can then look for other causes of shortness of breath."

The doctor gave a good explanation, Barbara noted, but she was determined to check on some more details on the Internet once she got home. "Is the test done here?" she asked Dr. Wilson.

"No, it's done at the cardiologist's office. There's one around the corner from here where I generally send my patients for a stress test."

With that, the doctor wrapped up the meeting after explaining how she would communicate the results of the tests and the need for follow-up appointments. Barbara and Susan walked out with some pamphlets about the various tests, appointment schedules, and directions to various test locations.

On the car ride home, Susan continued to find every reason why her problem could not be heart-related. Barbara saw no point in arguing when the test would reveal it one way or another, but she was curious about how doctors could tell if there were blockages with such a simple test.

When Exercise Was Considered "Dangerous"

In 1918, the electrocardiogram—or EKG as it's come to be known—was still evolving as a tool to look for heart diseases. Around this time, it was noted that an EKG monitored when the patient experienced chest pain showed some typical patterns that disappeared when the chest pain was relieved.[2] However, this observation was of limited use: The patient had to be having chest pain when they were in the limited area where this new technology was available. Therefore, these findings remained a curiosity without any real use in patient care.

During the late 1920s and early 1930s, some doctors noted that physical exertion or mental agony brought on chest pain in heart patients. Therefore, young doctors were taught that it was prudent for their patients to avoid any triggers that would provoke chest pain.[3] "Get some rest" became the standard advice given to patients with suspected heart disease.

Robert Bruce: Father of Exercise Physiology

Robert Arthur Bruce was born just outside of Boston on November 20, 1916. He grew up in Somerville and attended college locally, earning a bachelor of science from Boston University. He then went to the University of Rochester for medical school and later completed his advanced training. With his interest in and understanding of cardiology, he became the first director of the cardiology division at the University of Rochester in 1950.

Thinking about the heart, he considered how you would never buy a used car after just looking at it sitting idle in the dealer's lot, but you can learn a lot by taking it for a spin. Bruce then applied this logic to the human heart. If exercise evokes chest pain, and an EKG during chest pain helps detect heart problems, why not exercise the patient in the doctor's office and check their EKG at the same time?[4]

Initially, the only exercise routine that had been attempted in a doctor's office was the Master two-step test, during which the patient would repetitively climb up and down two nine-inch-high steps for ninety seconds. The doctor would attach the patient to the EKG machine before and after the exercise and make a recording.[5] Although this method had demonstrated the feasibility of exercise in heart patients, it was cumbersome and unreliable. It failed to gain widespread acceptance, because such a "one-size-fits-all" exercise proved both too little exertion to uncover any problems in some patients and too much exertion for others.

Bruce recognized these shortcomings and looked for better alternatives, turning to another form of standardized exercise.

Treadmills Are Dreadmills

Treadmills found their early use as a punishment for prisoners in England back in 1818. In later years, the practice was abandoned as inhumane.[6] However, in 1949, along with his team at Rochester, Robert Bruce began conducting experiments to assess respiratory function and heart rate using a standardized test that involved having his patients walk on a "motorized treadmill."

Bruce's team applied an EKG to the patient before the test and made continuous EKG recordings while the patient walked on the treadmill at a steady rate. They measured changes in heart rate and lung function before, during, and after a ten-minute exercise period. The team was able to safely perform the test on thousands of factory workers. Over time, they published reports on various changes in EKG patterns during the ten-minute exercise routine in those with and without heart disease. Despite the initial success, Bruce was keen to improve upon the test.

He realized that instead of a steady exertion, increasing the patient's workload might also increase the stress on the heart and reveal heart conditions with improved accuracy. Patients who had more blockages would show EKG changes early at low stress and would not have to be exercised to the next stage. For those with fewer blockages, the EKG would only detect a problem at high stress.

During the 1950s, Bruce refined his protocol into a multistage test with increasing stress. In 1963, he reported that his increased-workload protocol improved the accuracy of diagnosis without compromising patient safety.[7] This soon became known as the Bruce protocol and became the standard exercise protocol. Thousands of patients have undergone this mode of stress test over the intervening years. The safety of the test as well as changes in the EKG, blood pressure, and heart rate that may suggest the possibility of heart disease were well established by Bruce in subsequent reports. His findings are still used today, more than half a century later.

Through his pioneering work, Robert Bruce established himself as the father of exercise cardiology.

New and Improved Stress Tests

In addition to the EKG, other methods of "visualizing" the heart were combined with the stress test. Radioactive dyes injected through an IV line make their way to the heart muscle through the heart arteries. When the dye reaches the heart muscle, it lights up on the camera, indicating that there is an unblocked heart artery bringing blood to the heart muscle. On the other hand, if there is a blockage, the heart muscles will not receive blood supply, and a defect will be detected in the picture. By adding the radioactive dye to the EKG component of the stress test, the accuracy of the stress test is improved.

Another enhancement is the use of ultrasound of the heart called an *echocardiogram*. With this test, in addition to the EKG, ultrasound of the heart is performed before and after exercise. If there is low blood flow at the peak of exercise, the echocardiogram will show a defect in the pumping function of the heart muscles and help detect blockages.

These tests have enabled cardiologists all over the world to detect blockages in the heart arteries of millions of patients. After an abnormal stress test indicates possible blockages in the heart arteries, the patient usually undergoes a more definitive yet invasive procedure called *cardiac catheterization*.[8] In this test, doctors pass a tube through the leg or arm into the heart arteries. They then inject dye directly into the heart arteries and look at the location and extent of blockages. Based on the results, either medications alone, medications with bypass surgery, or medications with angioplasty is recommended as treatment.

On the other hand, if the stress test is normal, the chance of blockages in the heart arteries is very low. The normal stress test helps doctors rule out heart blockages as the cause of patient's symptoms without performing any further invasive procedures.[9] This saves numerous patients from having to undergo invasive procedures with potentially serious complications.

The stress test has helped save thousands of lives by detecting coronary disease, but it has probably saved many more lives and reduced costs heavily by excluding coronary disease without the need for an invasive procedure.

Susan's Smooth Recovery

Three months had passed since the stress test indicating the possibility of blockages in Susan's heart arteries. These blockages had later been confirmed by a cardiac catheterization.

Susan had many blockages in several of her heart arteries, and she was recommended bypass surgery. After getting identical opinions from two different cardiologists, she underwent the surgery. She had recovered well and successfully completed six weeks of physical-therapy rehab before returning to walking with Barbara.

Barbara found herself almost giddy with joy on the day they resumed their routine. "It's good to have our walks back, Susan."

"You're telling me! I'm so glad to put all that behind me and get back to my life. I will never complain about having a boring, unexciting, routine life. I was yearning to get back to this."

"Isn't that the truth? At our age, boring is good!"

Both relieved, the friends shared a good laugh.

"I am kind of disappointed I missed out on walking this summer; winter isn't far away," Susan lamented.

"Well, as the doctor said, the bypass surgery has probably increased your life span. You've probably gained a few summers by losing this one," Barbara pointed out, always the glass-half-full type.

They walked for about thirty minutes, which Susan was able to manage just fine. She was not back to her old self just yet, but she was definitely better than right before the surgery.

Over the next month and a half, Susan regained all of her energy, and she was back to walking as she had in the past. The friends enjoyed the mild autumn temperatures, but the holiday season proved hit-or-miss for their walking routine, what with family visits or travels. However, once the New Year arrived, they were keen to get back to their regular habit and lose the holiday weight.

Wishing for the Same Old, Same Old

"Good to be back, isn't it?" Susan spoke for both of them as they sat down for coffee after one of their daily walks.

"Yes, great to be back. I enjoy visiting family, but the travel is terrible these days," Barbara replied.

"It must have been nice to visit your son in New Jersey," Susan pointed out.

"Yes, and my old neighbors and friends. They all complain about the cold winter but continue to suffer through it. They talk about moving but never do."

"Did it snow a lot when you were there?" Susan inquired.

"Yes, we had tons of snow," Barbara responded.

"Oh, that couldn't have been fun! I used to hate the winters; I was cooped up inside every winter when I lived in Vermont. Did you get out much?"

"Yes, we bundled up and ventured out quite often, but I guess I'm no longer used to walking on the snow. I fell on an ice patch the last day I was there, and I'm still in pain and limping a little from the fall," Barbara revealed.

"Oh, dear! Are you okay to continue our walks? We can take a break if you like," Susan offered, though very reluctantly.

"No, I think I'll be fine in a couple days. It's nothing some ice and ibuprofen won't take care of." Barbara was determined to continue their routine now that she was back in town.

The Knee Problem Continues

Barbara's hopes of a quick recovery did not come to pass. She continued to limp for a couple of weeks, during which time her pain kept getting worse. After some resistance, she finally decided to go to her family doctor, who examined her knee and said something about feeling a click in her joint. He sent her for an MRI, which unfortunately showed a torn ligament. Barbara was referred to an orthopedic surgeon. The surgeon gave her the option of physical therapy for three months or knee surgery to repair the tear. Barbara felt most comfortable with the option of surgery. She would rather get it done and get back to her routine than spend three months trying physical therapy.

Quick surgery, quick recovery! she thought.

However, when she tried to schedule the surgery, she was asked to get clearance from a cardiologist first. Her insistence that "I don't have a heart condition" fell on deaf ears. They said something about safety, Barbara's age, how common heart disease is, blah, blah, blah . . . All this threw a wrench in Barbara's plan for a quick surgery and recovery. She was left with no choice but to get the clearance from the cardiologist. No clearance, no surgery, no recovery!

Barbara requested that Susan come along for her cardiologist appointment, as she had already been down this path. "It'll be better to have you along. I always get lost in all the medical jargon they use," she explained.

"Yes, it's another language altogether. Even their simple language stops making sense after a while!" Susan added.

"Have you heard about the patient from around here who suffered from a condition called *pholenfrometry*?"

"No, what is it? How on earth do you get something as serious-sounding as that?"

"I guess he fell from a tree!" Barbara winked, and the friends burst out laughing.

A Different Experience at the Doctor's Office

"So, I understand that you are planning to undergo knee surgery, Barbara," Dr. Shandra opened upon entering the room. His eyes shifted between Susan and Barbara, not sure who was the patient. He took a sip from his can of Diet Pepsi while waiting for a response.

Barbara spoke up. "Yes, the surgeon wants an okay from you first." It felt like she was here to be blessed before the surgery.

"Okay, so let's see . . ." Dr. Shandra scanned her chart. "You are seventy-two, right?"

Before Barbara could answer, he continued, "Do you have high blood pressure, diabetes, or any family history of heart disease?" His rapid speech made Barbara realize that he was in a rush.

"I take medicine for high blood pressure," was all Barbara could get out before Dr. Shandra started talking again.

"We don't have a cholesterol level for you . . . Are you a smoker?"

"No—quit when I was thirty-two." Barbara knew by now that she had to keep it short.

"Okay, so we'll check your cholesterol level and get a stress test and echocardiogram done. If all's clear, you can go through with surgery, no problem." Dr. Shandra kept nodding as if he were agreeing to his own recommendations. He was out the door before Barbara or Susan could ask any questions.

Barbara was devastated. She had been planning to get the surgery in a week or so and move on with her life, but it was going to be pushed back with all these tests. She didn't understand any of this. When she had gone with Susan to her doctor, they had known there was a problem, and the tests were necessary to diagnose the cause of her breathing difficulty. However, Barbara wasn't having any of those problems, so why did she need all these tests? It seemed like a waste of time to her, but what choice did she have? *No test, no clearance, no surgery, no recovery!*

Barbara had always been a get-it-done gal. After the initial shock and disappointment wore off, she decided to forge ahead so she could get the tests over with. She requested the earliest appointment she could get and even asked to remain on the standby list in case there was a cancellation sooner. The next week, they got her in for the echocardiogram, and the week after that, the stress test. Of course, she could not walk on her bad knee, so they did a "chemical" stress test, which apparently mimicked the changes observed during exercise and gave the doctors the same information. She got a call from the doctor's office the next day.

One and Done, or Is There More?

"Hi, Barbara! This is Linda from Dr. Shandra's office. How are you doing?"

"I'm well." Barbara was apprehensive.

"Barbara, your echocardiogram was normal, so your heart pumps well and your valves are working well."

There was a pause, and Barbara was quick to fill the silence. "Great! So Dr. Shandra will clear me for the surgery and I can go ahead and schedule it, right?"

"Well, unfortunately, the stress test was not normal. Dr. Shandra feels that you should come in for a cardiac catheterization to make sure there are no blockages before he clears you for the surgery," Linda said.

Barbara was dismayed and couldn't hide it. "But I haven't had any chest pain, breathing difficulty, or sweating. I eat a healthy diet, and I used to walk every day. How can I have blockages and not have any problems?" she asked, trying to argue her way out of it.

"Sometimes these blockages can be a silent killer. Heart disease kills thousands of people. It's better to be safe and get it checked out. At your age, there's always a small risk of heart blockages, and they can raise their ugly heads during surgery. Dr. Shandra often talks about the patient he saw few years back who had a heart attack after the surgery even though she'd had no signs of heart disease before the surgery. With this test, we can be sure that you'll go through the knee surgery without problems. You're lucky that we have the technology to make sure all's well."

Linda was clearly trying to convince her of the value of the testing. Barbara wasn't quite convinced, but she realized there was no talking her way out of this and went back into get-it-done mode.

"My friend Susan had a test where they put a tube in her heart arteries and injected dye into it. I think they took some pictures and saw blockages. Is this what you're talking about?"

"Yes, exactly!" Linda then discussed where and when to show up and what to expect.

Having accompanied Susan to these tests six or seven months ago, Barbara remembered some of the routine. Her son was not able to fly out on such short notice, so Susan accompanied her. Her experience with these tests would be helpful in navigating the system, Barbara concluded.

Back with the Cardiologist

Although things were done a little differently with Barbara's cardiologist, the essence of the process was the same as it had been with Susan. Barbara was taken to the holding area and she changed into a patient gown. An IV was placed, and blood was drawn and tested.

Dr. Shandra came in, Diet Pepsi in hand. He talked to Barbara about the risks, and then she was wheeled off for the procedure. They said it would take forty-five minutes. Susan got a cup of coffee and waited in the family area. After the forty-five minutes had passed, time slowed down. Susan kept looking nervously at her watch. An hour passed, then an hour and a half, with no indication of what was taking so long.

At the two-hour mark, Susan asked the front desk to look into the delay. The secretary was very pleasant and helpful. She called someone and, after what seemed like an eternity, hung up the phone. She told Susan that they had just finished and that Dr. Shandra would be out to talk to her soon.

Ten minutes later, Dr. Shandra approached Susan. His downcast gaze was not reassuring, and she suddenly feared that Barbara might also need bypass surgery.

"I am sorry it took so long. All is well. Barbara is doing fine." Then Dr. Shandra sighed. "We were done with the initial portion very quickly. However, while taking some final pictures, one of the arteries was damaged, and we had to put in a stent urgently," he said, his voice a little softer and more timid than it had been before the procedure. "She's fine now," he reassured Susan again.

"Stents? So, you found blockages?" Susan was confused about what he was trying to say.

"No, no blockages. Her heart arteries were clear."

"So, the stent had to be placed because . . ." Susan wasn't quite sure but had a premonition that something was being kept from her.

"One of the heart arteries suffered a dissection—a tear—when we were taking pictures, so we had to put in a stent," Dr. Shandra tried to clarify.

"Was that why she had the abnormal stress test?"

"No, her stress test was wrong. She had no blockages, but when we were taking the pictures of her heart arteries, the catheter caused a tear to her heart artery." He tried to mimic the tear with his hands, but the sign was lost on Susan. "With this tear, the blood flow through the artery stopped, so we put in the stent. It was a complication of the procedure. I am sorry about that."

"The stress test was wrong?" Susan clarified, surprised.

"Yes, the stress test suggested that there could be blockages; however, there were none," Dr. Shandra agreed.

"And the stress test should have been normal if she had no blockages?" Susan tried to make sure that she understood all of this.

"Yes, but it's not a perfect test. It sometimes indicates blockages when there are none," Dr. Shandra explained. As if to compensate for not mentioning any of this before, he repeated, "It is not a perfect test," shrugging his shoulders.

"Hmm . . . Would she have been better off without getting the stress test?" Susan questioned, her face betraying nothing.

"In hindsight, one can wonder about that, but I think it's better to get a stress test before any surgery. I had a patient few years back who had no heart condition but went through surgery and had a heart attack afterward. Based on my experience, I believe that it's better to know about the heart problems before surgery rather than be surprised afterward."

Susan's silence spoke volumes about her continued doubt. She kept her head down, avoiding Dr. Shandra's gaze.

"The nurses will call you in twenty minutes or so to visit Barbara." Without another word, Dr. Shandra rushed off. He did not want to spend any more time talking to Susan. He knew that as it was he would have to explain this to Barbara once she came off of the sedation.

As If That Weren't Bad Enough

The next day, Barbara was to be discharged from the hospital. Her son would be flying in that evening, so Susan was going to drive her home.

Dr. Shandra's assistant came in to discharge Barbara and explain the dos and don'ts after the procedure. She went over all the medication that she would have to take from this point on, giving special emphasis to the blood thinner.

"You cannot miss this one medication for a year. Not one day, not one dose. If you do, your stent could get blocked off, and you could have a heart attack." The assistant spoke with gravity and could not have been clearer.

"Okay." Barbara had come to terms with the doctors and their system at this point and felt like she had no control over the situation. It was a roller-coaster ride she would just have to go along with and follow their instructions on. If she wanted the knee surgery, she had to, she told herself.

"While you're on the blood thinner, do not use Motrin or Advil or any of those types of painkillers," the assistant said, continuing her spiel.

"But I've been using Advil for my knee pain; the surgeon said I can use it until my surgery." Barbara wanted to make sure she was safe to use them, and the news worried her.

"What surgery?" The assistant was puzzled.

"My knee surgery. That's what started this whole process; I needed clearance for knee surgery, so they did the stress test, and then . . ." Barbara shrugged, not wanting to mention the complication of the procedure again. She was always surprised that in health care the right hand didn't know what the left hand was doing.

"You should take Tylenol," the assistant suggested.

"It doesn't do anything for my pain. I'll see if the surgery can be done sooner, and then I won't have to worry about it." It would be difficult, but Barbara thought it might be the best way to resolve the issue.

"That won't be possible. They should not do any surgery that is not an absolute emergency for a year after you get this stent."

The assistant's words felt like a sucker punch to Barbara, who was too stunned to say anything. Susan, also stunned, wanted to be sure there was a good reason for this new instruction.

"No surgeon performs elective surgeries while a patient is on this blood thinner, because the bleeding could be disastrous. The recommendation is to hold off on any nonemergency surgery for a year. You'll be okay to stop the blood thinner after a year, and then you can get the surgery." The assistant casually mentioned a year as if it were a day. It felt like an eternity to Barbara.

"And no painkillers until then either?" Susan asked. She couldn't believe that all of Barbara's options were being taken away. This was going to be a long year. There was going to be no clearance, no surgery, and no relief for Barbara, even after all of this.

"The inflated fear of heart blockages has now created this real problem of stents and blood thinners. It's as though I was worried about getting into an accident while driving on the freeway, so I chose to walk on it instead and got run over. The treatment is worse than the disease!" Barbara exclaimed.

The room fell silent.

Stress Tests: A National Epidemic; Who Needs a Stress Test Prior to Surgery, and Who Gets It?

The stress test has proven to be a useful medical tool for a number of decades and over time has become more widely used. From the 1990s to the 2000s, there was a substantial increase in the rate of recommendation for stress tests to be performed before any surgery. However, widespread use can easily become reckless use.

In the 1990s, one in fifty-seven patients receiving a stress test didn't need it. By the 2000s, this had increased to one in fifteen patients. In some cases, as many as one out of two patients were undergoing unneeded stress tests.[10] These unnecessary stress tests delay the more necessary procedures and increase the patient's stay in hospital.[11] They also lead to further unnecessary testing if the initial stress test is abnormal, as in Barbara's case.

Does It Happen in Patients Who *Do Not* Need Surgery?

It is by no means only presurgery that the stress test is excessively ordered. Overall, the use of the stress test has increased, up by as much as 50 percent in frequency from the 1990s to the 2000s.[12]

Thanks to the ready availability of a stress test with radioactive dye, this technology is used too frequently. In the 1990s, only half of stress tests were performed with radioactive-dye injections. However, by the 2000s close to 90 percent of tests also used radioactive dye. It is estimated that one-third of these tests were not medically necessary. All the radiation exposure through these unnecessary tests causes 491 additional cancers per year. In addition, the economic cost of these tests is estimated at about 501 million dollars annually.[13]

The other downside to these unnecessary tests is that they lead to further unnecessary procedures. As in Barbara's case, one in eleven patients tested as abnormal on the stress test and ten normal. Interestingly, out of those that tested positive and underwent catheterization, two of the three did not have a significant blockage.[14] This reflects Barbara's situation, where the stress test wrongly suggested an abnormality. Some of these patients, like Barbara, were unfortunate, and suffered complications from a resulting procedure they did not need.

Who Gets These Tests?

The idea of any testing is to assess patients who are at risk of a poor medical outcome—such as heart attacks, stroke, or death—and to change the course of this "natural" phenomenon. Those patients with greater than a six in a thousand chance of death per year benefit from further testing, but studies have often shown that a number of patients who actually undergo the stress test are at very low risk of poor medical outcome. Their average rate of death is close to two in a thousand, and they should never undergo a stress test. Patients at such a low risk get no benefit from it and in fact are likely to be harmed by the stress test itself. And yet in some parts of the United States there is a four-fold prescription of stress test compared to other regions, all of which leads to little benefit and much harm.

What about an Annual Stress Test after Stent Placement or Bypass Surgery?

Even among patients who have had previous stent placement or bypass surgery, subsequent "routine" annual stress testing has not been shown to alter the patient's longevity.[15] One out of two patients had repeated the stress test within two years of these stents and bypass surgeries.[16] After having these "routine" stress tests, more than one in ten patients were recommended a repeat stent or bypass surgery. However, patients who had the repeat stent or bypass did not have any increase in longevity or decrease in heart attacks compared to those who never got a "routine" stress test. The tests led to more tests and more procedures but at no benefit to the patient.[17] Therefore, even among patients with a previous heart condition, the stress test does not yield any benefit when there are no symptoms and can instead lead to unnecessary stents or bypasses.

Why Does This Happen?

Many health-care advocacy groups have teased out the reasons why there is increasing use of these tests despite overwhelming scientific evidence that they do not always help. In the United States, we have a fee-for-service model in health care. This means professionals get paid for the services provided. If a physician or physician's office performs a stress test, they get paid for doing so. This leads to a considerable incentive for physicians to perform an increased number of costly procedures, even if they are not needed.[18] Tellingly, the number of stress tests performed decreased only after the reimbursement for these tests decreased in 2005.

Furthermore, when a surgeon sends a patient to a cardiologist's office for a stress test, even if it is unnecessary, cardiologists find it difficult to refuse the procedure. A denial of the test may make the surgeon feel challenged or offended, prompting them to start sending patients to other cardiologists for testing. Such a fear of loss of business may play a significant role in the overuse of needless stress tests.

Additionally, medicolegal liability plays some role in the overuse of testing, since physicians feel that by documenting a normal stress test they may avoid a lawsuit if the patient has a poor outcome from the surgery.[19] Some physicians, such as Dr. Shandra in Barbara's case, may have had or heard about a patient who had issues after a surgery. A negative case stands out in their mind even though thousands of others do well without a stress test. This is a cognitive error called *availability bias*, which drives physicians to judge the likelihood of a disease based on how easy it is to recall a particular case.[20] In Dr. Shandra's case, the one patient who had suffered an unexpected heart attack after surgery makes him overly cautious, though thousands of his other patients may have gone through such a surgery without a hitch.

The Agents of Change

In recent times, there has been increasing recognition of this overuse of stress tests. The American College of Cardiology has participated in a campaign called Choose Wisely, which aims to reduce the number of stress tests performed among patients in whom there is no scientific evidence of benefit from such test. These include patients with no symptoms of new blockages in the heart arteries, regardless of previous heart condition. The campaign aims to impress upon physicians the need to refrain from performing stress tests among patients who are undergoing low-risk surgery, such as knee or hip surgery, since stress tests have no beneficial effects on these patients.[21] It can also be harmful, as in Barbara's case.

APPENDIX

What Is a Stress Test?

A *cardiac stress test* is used to determine if there is low blood flow to the heart. In most cases, a patient exercises either on a treadmill or on a bike, with gradually increasing difficulty. During this process, the patient's EKG, blood pressure, and heart rate are checked. Changes in the EKG that occur with exercise may indicate low blood flow in the heart arteries. If this happens, the doctor may want to do other tests to verify that this is indeed the case.

At times, the doctor may recommend that the patient get a stress test with radioactive dye. In this case, a technician will inject dye and get pictures of the patient's heart before the exercise. The patient will then be asked to exercise, and the technician will inject dye once again at the peak of exercise. After exercise, another set of pictures is taken. The before and after pictures of your heart help the doctor better detect if there are blockages in the heart arteries.

Occasionally, instead of the nuclear dye the doctor may choose to get an echocardiogram done before and after the exercise. This test also adds value in helping detect blockages in the heart arteries.

If the patient is not able to walk or exercise for whatever reason, the doctor will order a chemical stress test. Here, the technician injects radioactive dye at rest and gets pictures of the patient's heart. Then, they give a medicine, followed by more radioactive dye, and take pictures once again. The doctor will then look at the before and after pictures to determine if there may be blockages in the heart arteries.

Why Do I Need Either the Echocardiogram or Radioactive Dye with My Stress Test?

The EKG part of the stress test is helpful, but it misses heart blockages in a certain number of people. A radioactive dye or echocardiogram decreases the chance of missing these blockages. In some patients, the EKG at rest is such that EKG during and after exercise cannot be accurately interpreted. In these patients, echocardiogram or radioactive dye adds value to the stress test.

I Have No Symptoms like Chest Pain, Shortness of Breath, Dizziness, Increased Sweating, Jaw Pain, or Left-Arm Pain. Do I Need a Stress Test Just Because I Am Over Sixty Years of Age?

If you have no symptoms, there is very little need for a stress test. The actions that will be taken from the results of the stress test are not going to prolong your life under these circumstances. As a matter of fact, you have more chance of being harmed by the test than being helped by it.[22]

I Need Surgery. Do I Need to Go Through a Stress Test to Make Sure I'm Safe?

Let's answer a few questions to try to find the solution:

- Can you climb a flight of stairs or walk up a hill?
- Can you run a short distance?
- Can you do heavy work around the house, like scrubbing floors or lifting or moving heavy furniture?
- Is it possible for you to do yardwork, including raking leaves, weeding, or pushing a power mower?
- Can you have sexual relations?
- Do you play golf or go bowling or dancing?
- Do you play doubles tennis?
- Can you throw a baseball or football?
- Do you participate in strenuous sports, like swimming, singles tennis, football, basketball, or skiing?

If you answered yes to any of these and have no symptoms, *you do not need a stress test.*[23]

If you answered no to all of these questions, answer these:

- Do you have kidney problems?
- Do you have known blockages in the heart artery for which you have had a stent or bypass surgery?
- Do you have to take insulin for diabetes?
- Have you had a stroke?
- Do you have congestive heart failure or a weak heart?
- Are you undergoing surgery of the blood vessels in the chest, abdomen, or above the pelvis?[24]

If you answered yes to more than one of these, you are at risk for heart problems around the time of high risk surgery.

The type of surgery also plays a role in determining if you need stress test prior. Low risk surgery, even when some of the answers are yes, does not merit pre-operative stress test.

I Have Had Blockages in the Heart Arteries and Have Had a Stent and/or Bypass Surgery to Treat Them. Do I Need a Stress Test Every Year?

If you have no symptoms, you will not benefit from a stress test. The chances are that either the stress test or the tests that could follow it may harm you more than help you.

As a result, the American College of Cardiology does not recommend routine stress tests.[25]

If I Have Been Having Chest Pain, Do I Need a Stress Test?

It depends. If your doctor determines that the cause is likely to be heart-related and you have other risk factors for heart disease, a stress test may be recommended. If your doctor determines that your chest pain is not similar to that associated with heart disease and you do not have any risk factors, they may not perform a stress test. You may use the calculator at https://qxmd.com/calculate/calculator_287/pre-test-probability-of-cad-cad-consortium to get a preliminary idea if you will benefit from stress test.

Are There Some Other Conditions under Which Stress Tests May Be Performed?

Yes—there are some rare situations, such as exercise-triggered heart-rhythm problems, for example, where a stress test may be helpful. Under these rare circumstances it may be worthwhile, following your doctor's advice on these tests.

What Happens If My Stress Test Is Abnormal?

If there are abnormalities found on the stress test, your doctor may recommend a *coronary angiogram*, which is also known as *cardiac catheterization*. This is the gold standard for figuring out whether or not there are blockages in the heart artery. Under certain specific circumstances, your doctor may also recommend a special CT scan to detect blockages in the heart arteries.

I Was Able to Walk on the Treadmill for More than Ten Minutes. Is That a Good Sign?

This is an excellent sign. Exercise duration is one of the strongest predictors of how long you will avoid a heart condition. The longer you can keep going on the treadmill, the less likely you will die of coronary artery disease soon—even if you currently have heart disease.[26]

**If My Stress Test Is Normal, Does That Mean I Will Not Have
a Heart Attack?**

A normal stress test tells you that your chances of a heart attack are low but
not zero. You will occasionally hear news stories of patients dying of heart attacks after having normal stress tests. However, this does not mean that a stress
test is unreliable. It only means that these rare cases still happen. A normal
stress test is usually a highly reliable test.

2

Cardiac Catheterization: That's Our Protocol

We fail more often because we solve the wrong problem than because we get the wrong solution to the right problem.

—Russell L. Ackoff[1]

CARDIAC CATHETERIZATION, AKA HEART CATH, CORONARY ANGIOGRAM

A Fighting Spirit

Carl had always been a fighter. That was how he had made it through life. He had lost his father at an early age, but right out of high school he had enrolled in the army and was deployed to Vietnam. In his second year of service, his unit was ambushed, and he was injured by a bomb that had exploded a few feet from him. He survived but lost his spleen and one kidney. After returning home, he went to college on the GI Bill, later becoming a realtor and real estate investor during the housing boom in Houston.

Over his lifetime, Carl had lived through two bankruptcies, a divorce, and the death of his young son. He had always made it through these tough times and seemed to take it all in his stride. "This too shall pass," was his response to everything fate threw at him. After the storm passed, he would remember only the good times and none of the difficulties, seemingly gifted with a selective memory.

The first six months of this past year had been tough; he had undergone che-motherapy and then radiation therapy for stomach cancer. Every other month he was driving all the way across the city to see his oncologist—the doctor who specialized in treating his cancer. However, when the family gathered around him on his eighty-fifth birthday, there was no place for cancer. His two sons, daughter, and seven grandchildren, the light of his life, all sang, danced, and shared the many wonderful memories they'd made with him over the years.

While he enjoyed the break, he soon wanted to get back into his routine. However, two weeks after his birthday, he was struggling. His regular visits to the gym had to be shortened, and sometimes skipped entirely, due to fatigue and breathing difficulties. He was finding it increasingly hard to continue his usual forty-five minutes on the elliptical machine and was getting winded easily. After struggling for a week, he decided to work on his strength and tone, taking up weight training. His family doctor had told him that this was critical for his bone health and balance. What Carl could not perform in cardio, he would achieve through strength training.

The Struggle Worsens

A week or so went by, but Carl's breathing and stamina did not return to normal. As a matter of fact, the weight training seemed to be giving him added aches and pains. He tried to ignore them, because he had been advised to avoid painkillers, as they placed too much of a burden on his solitary kidney. Two weeks later, when the fatigue and muscle aches continued and his breathing did not improve, he decided to call his family doctor.

"Can I get in to see Dr. Chappell? I am a regular patient of hers," Carl asked the receptionist on the phone.

"Yes, we can get you in. Let me see when Dr. Chappell's next open slot is," the receptionist said. "Oh, before I do that, what's the reason for your visit?"

"I've been kind of out of breath lately. When I exercise, I get winded easily," Carl said.

"Oh, that's not good," the receptionist said. She was pleasant enough, but the words felt empty and scripted. Carl heard the clickety-clack of the keyboard as she typed. "Do you have any chest pain, Carl?"

"I have aches and pain all over, so you could say that," Carl tried to explain.

"Is that a yes for chest pain, Carl?" she asked, looking for a yes-or-no answer.

"Yes, I guess," Carl responded with exasperation, not sure that all they were asking could be answered with a simple yes or no.

"Okay, let's see . . ." There was more clicking of the computer, and then she continued, "Carl, because of your chest pain, we have to get you in today, or you have to go to the emergency room. It's our protocol. Can you come in today to see someone in the clinic?"

Carl was surprised that there was a protocol to get him seen sooner. He had always assumed the processes at doctor's offices delayed rather than expedited things. "Yes, I can come in today."

"Dr. Chappell is not around today, but I can get you in to see one of her assistants," said the receptionist. "Sean has an opening at 3 p.m. Can you come in at three?"

"Yes, but I would rather see Dr. Chappell. She knows me well." Carl offered only gentle resistance, knowing there was not much room for negotiation at the doctor's office.

"Dr. Chappell is not here today, and because of your chest pain, we have to get you in ASAP. Can I put you in with Sean for today?" the receptionist persisted. She was trained to follow protocols, not patient preferences.

"Yeah, sure." Carl realized the futility of trying to argue and went with the flow.

"Okay then, we'll see you at three. Don't forget to bring your medications with you," the receptionist added, ending the conversation.

When Carl went to the gym later that morning, he felt glad they could get him in that day. His breathing was getting worse.

At the Doctor's Office

Dr. Chappell's office wasn't too far from Carl's house. When he arrived fifteen minutes before his appointment, he was told that Sean was running late. "He's having one of those days!" the receptionist smiled.

By 3:30 p.m., Carl was beginning to wonder if they would be able to take him in before the office closed at 4 p.m. or if he would have to make another appointment, but he patiently continued to wait. At 3:40 p.m., the assistant came out and called his name. Hopefully he would soon get some resolution to his breathing issues.

Inside the exam room, the assistant checked his blood pressure and pulse. "Have you lost some weight recently?"

"A little, not much," Carl replied.

"Okay. Has any of your medication changed since last time?" the assistant asked.

"No. They're all the same," he responded. He wanted to get this done so that he could be seen.

"Have you brought your medications?"

"No, but you must have them in your computers," he answered, as he always did.

"Alright, I'll look it up. Sean should be in soon," the assistant called over her shoulder as she walked out.

Within five minutes, Sean showed up. Dr. Chappell always shook Carl's hand and sat down, but Sean stood tall over him.

"You were an add-on today, Carl . . . Davis?" he said, reading from the chart, "And you're here for shortness of breath and chest pain, is that correct?"

"Yes. When I go to the gym, the shortness of breath becomes bothersome. I used to exercise for forty-five minutes at a time, but not anymore. I'm lucky to get in ten."

"And you're also having chest pain?" Sean asked.

"Yes—I have aches all over, including my chest." He felt rushed. It seemed Sean only wanted a yes or no answer.

"How long have you been having chest pain?" Sean asked, his speech clipped.

"About seven days."

"With exercise?"

"Well . . . yes. As a matter of fact—" Carl wanted to explain that his aches and pains had started after he'd begun weight training, but Sean quickly moved on to the next question. The visit felt too focused on his chest pain.

After another three minutes of quick-fire questions, Sean left. Within a minute, a doctor came in.

"Hello! I'm Dr. Johnstone, one of Dr. Chappell's partners. So, you're having chest pain with exercise, which is new?"

"Yes, that is true—" Carl felt like he should clarify that his bigger worry was the fatigue and breathing difficulty, but before he could, Dr. Johnstone started talking again.

"This is serious, Carl. At your age having a cholesterol problem as you do and now this chest pain is very concerning."

Carl was surprised at how quickly his shortness of breath and bodily aches and pains had been converted to chest pain. But before he could interrupt, Dr. Johnstone dropped a bombshell.

"We're going to send you to the hospital. This may be a sign of blockages in the heart arteries, which are not uncommon among men your age. I notice that you used to be a smoker." He only waited for a nod from Carl before continuing. "That adds further risk. This could be a serious issue. At the hospital, they'll perform a couple tests to look into the blockages of the heart arteries. Okay?" he concluded, leaving the room before Carl could ask any questions.

Someone wants to beat the 5 o'clock traffic! Carl thought.

Chest-Pain Protocol at the Hospital

Before he knew it, Carl was on a hospital bed, and swarms of people were coming at him for blood tests and to start IV lines. A young doctor came in and told him that Dr. Johnstone had called to say Carl was having heart trouble.

"Well, I had breathing difficulties when I was exercising—" Carl tried to explain.

"Yes, I have the notes from Dr. Johnstone here. He mentions that you experience angina. And, yes, he does mention your dyspnea with exercise, but you're otherwise healthy. You had splenectomy in the past and are a smoker, correct?"

"I was a smoker many years ago," Carl clarified, offering an answer to the only part of the jargon he understood. "Decades back," he emphasized. On more than one occasion, he wanted to mention his cancer, but he assumed that they would have it in their computer. Besides, no one seemed to have any time to hear the details—they were all focused on the chest pain.

The young doctor examined him and left, returning after fifteen minutes. "I talked to my attending physician, and he has talked to the cardiologist. The blood work shows that you are not having a heart attack right now, so there's no emergency, but we will do a heart cath tomorrow morning. You'll be NPO after midnight. We will get you to sign the paperwork," he continued. The technical language was foreign to Carl.

"What's it for?" Carl asked, trying to get some information.

"You're having chest pains with exercise, which could be due to blockages in the heart arteries," the young doctor answered. "In situations like this, we always do the heart cath. This is routine."

"I think the chest pain is muscle pain. I have aches and pains all over my body. I think they may be due to weight training," Carl said, finally bringing up his concerns.

"Still, we'd better make sure it isn't your heart. The cardiologist was concerned enough to schedule you first thing in the morning," the young doctor said, clearly trying to justify his approach.

"Will someone talk to Dr. Chappell about this? I want to make sure she's okay with it; she's known me for years."

"We'll let her know," the young doctor reassured him, avoiding his gaze.

When the doctor left, Carl was in a daze. Just a few hours before, he had been out and about, having the same aches and pains he'd had for two weeks. Now tests were coming at him almost out of nowhere! Later that day, the nurse came in to explain the procedure, talking about inserting a big IV line through his groin. They would put a tube near the heart through it, she said, and inject dye into the heart arteries. By looking at the X-ray while injecting the dye, they would check for blockages. She explained the procedure well. Carl was still not convinced he needed it, but he was nevertheless astounded by the technology. He wondered how it had come about.

A Pioneer, an Innovator, and Crazy, in Equal Measure

The heart has been the center of human attention for centuries, but the process of getting anywhere close to it has scared humankind through the ages. Early experiments were performed on animals by pioneers and on humans by renegades.

In the eighteenth-century, English clergyman Stephen Hales was famed for inserting pipes into a horse's veins to measure blood pressure—a practice that quickly encouraged him and others to repeat it with different animals and better instruments. Despite this, doing anything similar in humans was widely considered lunacy.[2]

By the early twentieth century, X-ray machines had been invented and popularized. And not long after, young German physician, Werner Forssmann, had become convinced that there was an advantage to injecting medication close to the heart and that X-ray technology would be extremely helpful in guiding catheters to the heart. During this period, it was commonly believed that touching the human heart with catheters would kill the patient, so when Werner suggested this to his supervisor he was forbidden from trying it on patients. Even Werner's offer to experiment on himself was instantly denied.

The surgical nurse had access to the instruments that Werner required, and he talked her into doing a minor procedure using them. However, in the middle of the "routine" procedure, the nurse realized that Werner planned to carry out an altogether different one and refused to cooperate. Werner tied her to the operating table, put a catheter in his own vein, and pushed it forward. In his own words, "I only perceived some sensation of warmth . . . there was no pain. I only felt warm sensation behind the clavicle . . . I checked the position radiologically by climbing from the OR to the radiology department."[3] He took X-ray pictures to prove that the catheter was actually close to the heart, and his own survival proved the safety of contact with the heart.

He published his work, which went on to inspire others but got him fired from his job. He continued to work with catheters, except as a urologist, not a cardiologist. While his publication inspired others, Werner himself remained unknown and unsung. He fought in World War II, was taken prisoner, and on his release worked as a woodcutter before returning to work as a physician.

Those who came after him were inspired by his work and continued to finesse the procedure. The art and science he had pioneered continued to progress in the United States.[4]

Serendipity Befalls a Prepared Mind

Getting a catheter close to the heart with the help of X-rays was only half the battle. Blockages in the heart arteries had been recognized as the source of heart attacks and chest pain since the 1920s. During this period, there was a great deal of interest in confirming these blockages in patients with chest pain.[5] Early experiments in the 1930s and 1940s were conducted on dogs.[6] Scientists injected dye into the heart arteries of the dogs with catastrophic results. The injections triggered fatal heart rhythms, causing the dogs' deaths. As a result, it became widely believed that injecting dye into the heart arteries of humans would kill them also.[7]

At Cleveland Clinic in the 1950s, Dr. Mason Sones was working in the basement, assessing his patients for heart conditions with an X-ray machine. He and his staff were well aware of the dangers of injecting dye into the heart arteries, choosing to inject at high pressure within close proximity. They made treatment decisions based on the hazy pictures they saw with this technique. They yearned for clearer images but dared not venture closer to the heart arteries.

On October 30, 1958, Sones was assessing a young patient. As a senior physician, he observed off to the side while the training physician directly attended to the patient, ready to inject the dye while X-ray images were taken. Dr. Sones instructed the trainee to inject the dye while he observed on the X-ray machine. To everyone's horror, the tube close to the heart artery jumped inside and expelled the dye right into the artery, something that was to be avoided at all costs. Dr. Sones jumped up and grabbed a scalpel, ready to open the patient's chest to save him from certain death. The patient's heart stopped for five seconds . . . but then resumed beating as normal. He recovered to see Dr. Sones hovering over him with a knife in his hand.[8]

Entirely by accident, the team had debunked the myth that dye injection into the heart arteries is fatal. Learning from this experience, Dr. Sones started intentionally injecting dye into patients' heart arteries, becoming increasingly assured of the safety of the procedure. The clearer images obtained thereby helped the team make better decisions for their patients. They fine-tuned their procedure further and published their efforts after four years.[9] Physicians from around the world now came to observe and learn from them.

Improvement and Acceptance

Throughout the 1960s, many other modifications were made to the procedure. Preshaped catheters were designed to assist getting into the heart arteries easily and safely, and X-ray machines were modified to suit the procedure's requirements. The composition of the dye injected into the heart arteries was also improved, enhancing its safety for the human body and improving its visibility.[10]

The procedure has since emerged as the cornerstone of cardiac testing. It is the gold standard in detecting blockages in the heart arteries. Since 1958, tremendous progress has been made in cardiology thanks to accurate diagnosis of blockages in the heart arteries.[11] And this increased accuracy has in turn enhanced our knowledge of what symptoms correlate with the blockages and helped us distinguish between heart-related symptoms and non-heart-related symptoms. We can more accurately assess the risk factors for heart blockages, like smoking, diabetes, and lack of exercise.

This diagnostic test has also enabled us to figure out what treatment best benefits varying types of blockages. For example, a blockage in the main artery on the left side is better treated with bypass surgery, whereas a blockage on the right side alone would be better treated with medicine or stents. If there are many different blockages all over, you are better off with bypass surgery. Sones's test paved the way for the treatment of heart blockages by means of angioplasty and stents. One doctor's accident was humanity's salvation.

Carl's Diagnosis

The morning after being unceremoniously rushed to the hospital, Carl underwent his procedure. He was glad it would be over early so that he wouldn't have to go hungry all day. He slept through the procedure because of the medicine they gave him. Thirty minutes after the procedure, the cardiologist came to his bedside. "Sorry it took a little longer than expected. The good news is all your heart arteries look okay. There were minor blockages of up to 50 to 60 percent, but nothing that needs stents or a bypass. We took a lot of pictures to make sure."

"Oh, thank you, doctor." Carl was relieved.

"While we were doing the test on your heart arteries, we did see something in the lungs. We'll do a chest X-ray to make sure, but we should be able to send you home soon," the cardiologist said, not appearing too concerned.

"Do you think that may be causing my breathing problems?" Carl asked, trying to connect the dots.

"Yes, of course. Did you tell anyone about them?" the cardiologist asked.

"Well, I kept telling them about the shortness of breath and these muscle pains, but they kept focusing on chest pain."

"They should have started with a chest x-ray. I guess they just got anchored to the phrase *chest pain* and forgot everything else. This happens all the time; doctors focus on one thing and forget the bigger picture. I'm sorry this happened to you. We should probably right the ship and get a chest X-ray," he concluded quickly.

Carl was touched by this admission but kept wondering how physicians, who are supposed to be the smartest, could make such errors in thinking. *I guess we're all human, even the brightest among us,* he concluded.

They took Carl for a chest X-ray after a few hours. Within minutes of it, the young doctor came by. "We're seeing some spots on the lungs, and they're concerning. Have you been losing weight?"

"Some, but not as much as before. I mentioned it to the nurse when she was asking a bunch of questions yesterday." Carl was always surprised that hospitals and clinics never seemed to talk to one another.

"Hmm. What do you mean? How much weight are we talking about?" The young doctor looked perplexed.

"Well, before I ended my chemotherapy in January, I lost about twenty pounds in three months. Recently, I've lost maybe . . . five pounds?" Carl guessed.

"Chemotherapy? For what?" the young doctor said, shuffling through Carl's papers.

"For my stomach cancer. It must be on my chart . . . I had chemotherapy in January," Carl clarified.

"I don't see anything like that." The young doctor's voice almost sounded accusatory.

"My cancer doctor must have sent the notes! I had chemotherapy at their offices on Broadway." Carl's concern over an apparent lack of communication was confirmed once again. He wondered briefly if other fields were as chaotic as health care.

"No, we don't have anything here." The young doctor was visibly distressed now. He paused for a moment, then flatly adding, "We'll have to do a CT scan to see if the cancer has spread." It was almost as if he were talking about something as minor as the brake pads of a car wearing out.

Carl was stunned. *Could it be?* He had believed the chemotherapy would take care of it. How could it have spread? He had just finished chemo, and they'd said everything looked good. They hadn't even scheduled another appointment with his cancer doctor for two months!

Carl was upset and angry, but he didn't know at whom. Was it the young doctor in front of him, the health-care system in general, cancer, his helplessness, or God for putting him through all this?

Carl had the CT scan, during which they injected some more IV dye and got pictures. Carl was anxious for the results, but nobody came to let him know. All he found out from the nurse was that he was staying the night. He spent a sleepless night worrying about the cancer and wondering if it had spread. The darkness of the night often brought up dark thoughts for Carl, but they usually evaporated in the sunlight. Not this time.

Bad Manners and Worse News

The young doctor was the first to visit him in the morning, running through his routine of asking how Carl had been during the night and other formalities. He was avoiding the eight-hundred-pound gorilla in the room. Finally, Carl asked about the results of the CT scan.

"Well, there are indeed a few spots on the lungs. It could indicate that the cancer has spread, or it could be something else. We may have to do some tests to figure it out." Carl felt a flash of annoyance at this doctor's wishy-washy attitude but kept quiet as he continued, "We're going to get your cancer doctors to see you. They may be able to tell you more." The young doctor was clearly uncomfortable; it appeared that he wanted someone else to talk to Carl about it.

"They'll see me while I'm here? Or am I going home today?"

"No, I think we'll keep you here; we need to give you some IV fluids. The function of your kidneys is a little off, probably from the IV dye you received yesterday," he explained. "They'll come and see you sometime today."

Carl shrugged in response. He wanted to remind the young doctor that he had only one kidney, he had lost the other in the war, but refrained. He just wanted to be left alone now. The darkness of the night seemed to have returned.

Over the course of the day, several doctors came in, but the most critical discussion occurred when Dr. Chappell came by to see him. It seemed that they had communicated with her at last.

After the usual pleasantries, she came to the meat of the matter. "Carl, I have talked to everyone on the team. So much has been going on that you must be dizzy from all the activity!"

Carl smiled. It finally seemed that someone understood what he was feeling.

"Let me help you understand what's going on." She paused to make sure he understood that she was going to spell it out for him. "You had the heart cath with IV dye, followed quickly by a CT scan with IV dye. All that dye has hurt the only kidney you have. Hopefully, it will recover in a few days. More importantly, I am very sorry to tell you that the cancer has most likely spread to the lungs." She paused to gauge Carl's reaction but quickly realized he was too stunned to react.

"This is not good news," she went on. "We will have to have longer conversations with the cancer doctors. Together we can discuss where to go from here, what treatment plans are possible, which are reasonable, and what they may or may not add to your survival and quality of life." Her tone conveyed the gravity of the situation. "Do you want your children to be here when we have the discussion with the cancer doctors?"

"No, they live far away," Carl said simply. He could do with their support but didn't want to bother them.

"Okay. I'll see if the cancer doctors can come in tomorrow for a meeting, if that's okay with you," she said.

"Yes—the sooner, the better." Carl didn't want to spend any more time worrying about it than he had to.

"Okay, then." Dr. Chappell started to leave but paused, as if she had forgotten something. "Carl, I want to apologize for how it all unfolded in the clinic and the hospital. I wish I had been in the clinic to see you myself. None of this would have happened," she confessed.

"What do you mean?" He was confused.

"Well, I knew about your cancer. If it had been communicated to the team, they would have looked at the lungs first rather than jumping to the heart-artery blockages. If they hadn't unnecessarily worried about the heart arteries, we could have saved the trouble with the kidneys. We created this kidney problem for you, and I am so sorry," she said, placing a hand on Carl's shoulder.

Her honesty touched Carl. She had stepped out of the doctor's role and displayed her humanity. This permitted Carl to reveal his. At that moment, his calm collapsed, and he broke down. "I just wish you could take away the cancer. I'm so scared."

The Ease, Praise, and Rise of Procedures

A number of tools and techniques were introduced in the decades after the initial cardiac cath to make the procedure safe. With the widespread utility of the procedure, the training of an increasing number of cardiologists to perform them, and its lucrative reimbursement, the number of heart catheterizations dramatically increased. From about two hundred thousand procedures in 1979, the number of cardiac catheterizations performed almost tripled by 1986. It is estimated that by the year 2000, about 1.2 million procedures were performed in the United States annually.[12] The procedure continues to be extensively used in the twenty-first century.

The widespread utility of this procedure to all who need it should be a sure sign of progress, but the reckless application of such an invasive procedure could harm many. It begs the question: Does the increased number of procedures reflect an increased number of people needing it, or is it down to the imprudent application of a potentially dangerous yet easy and profitable procedure to patients who don't need it?

One way to assess whether the number of people having heart disease is increasing is to look at the trend of heart attacks in the country. The rate of heart attacks is indicative of how prevalent coronary artery disease is in our society, because if such coronary artery disease becomes more common, then there are more heart attacks. If there were an increased number of heart attacks, and, by extension, an increased number of people with coronary artery disease, the increased use of heart catheterization would be welcomed and justified.

Unfortunately, the number of heart attacks recorded over the last few years has not changed. This means heart disease is only as common today as it was in the 1980s and 1990s. However, the number of people who have been tested has increased rapidly. This is an indication that cardiac catheterization could be overutilized. Unlike in the past, we may be applying invasive and expensive tests to people who are unlikely to benefit from it.[13]

Zooming In

That cardiac catheterization is being overused is further confirmed by other reports. In a sample of the US population who underwent heart cath procedures across a four-year period starting in 2003, only one of the three was found to have significant blockages. The other two were subjected to the risks of the procedure without any benefit. Could the physicians have done a better job selecting candidates for the procedure and avoided unnecessary testing?

The simple answer, per the report, is yes! If the physicians had followed the scientific recommendation to not subject patients without cardiac symptoms to heart cath procedures, *one-third* of patients would not have undergone them.[14]

Furthermore, the risk factors for heart-artery blockages are well known. The typical symptoms of these blockages have also been well validated. When the researchers plugged patient information into these known risk predictors, they were able to predict which patients may have critical blockages in over three out of four cases. The information used by the researchers had been readily available to the physicians performing these reckless procedures. If they had used it, they could have avoiding subjecting a large number of patients to such an invasive procedure.[15]

Poor selection subjects more patients to the risk of complications without any potential benefit.

So, How Many Cardiac Catheterizations Are Unnecessary?

In several reports over the years, it has been estimated that an average of 25 percent of patients underwent these tests when they had no symptoms of coronary artery disease. There are parts of the country where this number rises to 75 percent despite ample information that patients without symptoms will not benefit from the procedure. When patients without symptoms of heart disease undergo testing and blockages are found, treatment with stents or bypasses does not improve longevity. However, in hospitals where unnecessary testing takes place, there is also an increased rate of stent placement or bypass surgery to treat detected blockages, despite the fact that these patients get no benefit and are occasionally even harmed by these treatments.[16]

Therefore, one can safely conclude that at least *25 percent or one in four patients* in this country undergoing a heart cath will derive no benefit from it.[17]

In the report mentioned above, researchers were able to predict heart disease accurately in 75 percent of patients based on the known patient information and the scientific evidence available. The doctors who ordered cardiac catheterization failed to take the available information into account, and so their accuracy rate was only 36 percent. If the doctors had paid attention to all the relevant information and married it with known scientific evidence, they could have avoided this invasive procedure in almost 40 percent of their patients.[18]

Overall, it appears that anywhere between *25 to 40 percent* of heart catheterizations performed in the country are unwarranted.

The More You Look, the More You See, the More You Treat

Another concern that comes with overuse of the heart cath is the potential for overestimating the blockages in the heart arteries.[19] Reporting of blockages is based on the subjective assessment of the cardiologist doing the procedure. In one out of every eleven patients, there is an overestimation of these blockages. If the cardiologist estimates the blockage to be 70 percent when it is only 60 percent, it could make a difference between the decision to treat with medication alone versus using stents and medication. Such an overestimation of blockages is thought to translate into a large number of patients receiving unnecessary stents (approximately one in ten) and even bypass surgery (one in six).[20] The concern is that patients who were not even candidates may get tested unnecessarily and then treated because of erroneous interpretation. Such overtreatment does not result in any increase in life span—not even by one day. Patients undergoing testing and treatment under such circumstances do not have improved quality of life compared to those who do not get such aggressive therapy. Furthermore, all of the tests and treatments have significant complication rates.

But There Must Be Some Benefit to These Techniques . . .

If a patient is having a heart attack, cardiac catheterization and stent would be absolutely essential, and lifesaving. However, in the years that follow a heart attack, it is medication that helps, not repeat procedures.

In parts of the country with a higher concentration of cardiologists and procedure rooms, patients receive more procedures in the first decade after heart attacks but do not do any better than patients who get the appropriate medication and no additional procedures. If a patient is treated with the proper medication, further procedures add little value to their care.[21]

APPENDIX

What Are Coronary Arteries?

Coronary arteries supply blood to the heart itself. The heart gets its own blood supply from two major blood vessels—the left main artery and right coronary artery. The left main artery divides further into two branches. These branches, along with the right coronary artery, form the three major arteries supplying blood to the heart (see figure 2.1).

As we age, plaque is deposited in the arteries. This creates blockages for blood flow to the heart muscles. Factors such as smoking, diabetes, high blood pressure, high cholesterol, or a family history of blockages in these arteries before the age of fifty-five can increase the rate of plaque buildup. Although good blood flow through these arteries is essential to keeping the heart muscle

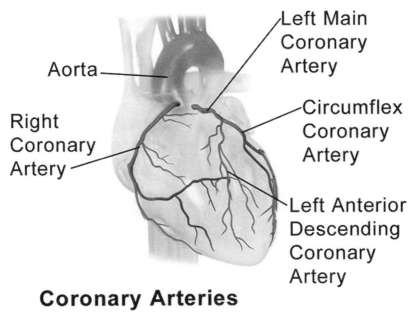

Coronary Arteries

Figure 2.1.   Coronary arteries
Blausen Medical Communication, Inc.

healthy and functioning at its best, the heart muscle can continue to function normally even with a 50 to 60 percent blockage (except in the left main artery, where anything more than 50 percent blockage is concerning).

When does one suspect blockages in the heart arteries?

The condition where a person has blockages in the heart arteries is called *coronary artery disease* (see figure 2.2). It develops over decades, and until the blockage is sufficient to decrease the flow of blood to the muscles of the heart, one may not have any symptoms.

When there is significant blockage in the heart arteries (more than 70 percent), one may experience the following symptoms:

Chest Pain or Chest Pressure

When associated with low blood flow in the coronary arteries, chest pain is called *angina*. It can feel like pressure or tightness or as if someone is standing

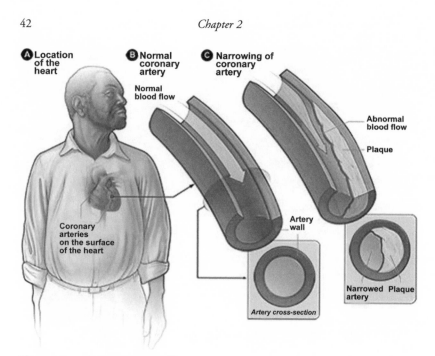

Figure 2.2.   Coronary artery disease
National Institutes of Health

on your chest. The patient may also experience pain in the neck or jaw. It occurs with physical or emotional stress and is relieved with rest and nitroglycerin. It can last five to fifteen minutes.

Shortness of Breath

Sometimes coronary artery disease may cause shortness of breath when the patient is under physical or emotional stress. It may be associated with chest pain.

If one has crushing chest pain that travels to the jaw or neck and persists for more than fifteen minutes, this may be a sign of a heart attack caused by complete blockage of one or more of the heart arteries. It may also cause shortness of breath, increased sweating, nausea, or vomiting. This pain does not go away with rest. This is a life-threatening situation, and emergency services should be called.

What Are the Risk Factors that Predispose One to Coronary Artery Disease? Who Is at Risk for Coronary Artery Disease?

Risk factors for coronary artery disease include

- Age: The chances of coronary artery disease increase with age.
- Gender: Men are at greater risk for developing coronary artery disease. Women are generally considered to be at low-risk before their menopause.
- Family history: A first degree relative having coronary artery disease at less than fifty-five years of age makes one more susceptible.
- Smoking: Smoking increases the chances of coronary artery disease. Exposure to secondhand smoke has a similar impact.
- Existing conditions: High blood pressure, high cholesterol, and diabetes greatly increase the risk of developing coronary artery disease.
- Obesity: Being obese increases your risk of the disease.
- Sedentary lifestyle: Inactivity can also increase your risk of heart disease.
- Unhealthy diet: Foods rich in saturated fat, trans fat, salt, and sugar can increase the chance of developing coronary artery disease.[22]

How Is a Diagnosis of Coronary Artery Disease Reached?

If you experience ongoing, unrelenting, crushing chest pain, it is critical to get to the ER. Here, an ECG would be the first test to rule out a heart attack. In addition, blood tests will be performed to check for chemicals in your blood that indicate a heart attack. If you are having a heart attack, you will likely to taken for immediate cardiac catheterization, with the possibility of putting in a stent. In such a life-threatening condition, a stent will be lifesaving.

However, if you present with a few days or weeks of chest pain or shortness of breath during exercise that subsides with rest, an ECG will be the initial test performed. It may or may not show abnormality regardless of whether you have coronary artery disease or not.

The key test will then either be a stress test or a cardiac catheterization (also known as a *coronary angiogram* or *heart cath*), depending on how likely the doctor believes your symptoms are coronary artery disease–related. The majority of the patients should go for a stress test; only a small minority with more than one of the above risk factors may be taken directly for cardiac catheterization.

It is not unusual to get a test called an *echocardiogram* during the process. This is an ultrasound of the heart. It helps doctors determine if your heart is pumping normally, if the heart muscles look normal and if there are any concerning valve leaks.

What Is a Cardiac Catheterization?

This is the gold standard for finding blockages in the coronary arteries. During this procedure, the doctor gains access into your artery in the arm or leg. From there, they thread a small, thin, flexible tube, called a *catheter*, into the heart arteries. They then proceed to inject dye into your arteries through this catheter while taking X-ray pictures. The dye flows through the coronary arteries and outlines them. If there is a blockage in the artery, there will be a visible narrowing on the X-ray.

Blockage in the heart artery is called *stenosis*. Doctors estimate the stenosis visually and give it percentages. The result of the test is reported as a percentage of stenosis in different coronary arteries—for example, 40 percent stenosis in the right coronary artery, 30 percent blockage in the left main artery, and so on. Depending on the degree of stenosis and number of blockages, the doctor will recommend no treatment, medicines, angioplasty (with stent) or bypass surgery.

Any stenosis of more than 50 percent in the left main artery or more than 70 percent in other coronary arteries may need more than medication. Stenosis of less than 70 percent in coronary arteries (other than the left main artery) is not considered critical and only requires medication and lifestyle changes.[23]

If Cardiac Catheterization Is the Gold Standard, Why Not Perform One for Everyone with Suspected Heart Disease?

There are many ways to assess whether there are blockages in the coronary arteries. Heart cath is an invasive procedure, and like all invasive procedures it has its risks. For every one hundred patients undergoing a heart cath, two will have major complications related to it.

These complications can include

- Heart attack related to the test
- Stroke
- Damage to the heart artery
- Puncture of a wall of the heart and blood seeping outside the heart (called a *tamponade*)
- Damage to the kidneys

- Infection
- Blood clots
- Death

Minor complications of the procedure may also arise:

- Bruising or blood accumulation in the arm or groin where the catheter was
- Damage to the artery where the catheter was inserted (*pseudoaneurysm*)
- Irregular heart rhythms (*arrhythmias*)
- Allergic reaction to the IV dye[24]

These risks may be of concern depending on your situation. If you have a high risk of blockages in the coronary artery, finding out about them will be helpful and in some cases lifesaving. However, if you do not have risk factors for coronary artery disease, the risks of the procedure outweigh any real benefit from it. In that case, the risks of the procedure are outweighed by benefits of the procedure.

If you are unfortunately at a stage in life where other diseases are taking their toll and expected life span is less than a few months, there is no benefit in doing this test to look for blockages.

If you do not have symptoms of chest pain or shortness of breath, the benefit of this procedure would be too small to undertake the risks. If a cardiac cath is recommended, you should consider seeking a second opinion from another doctor who won't be performing the procedure if you feel unsure. Ideally, this physician should not work in the same group as the one who first recommends the procedure; perhaps find a cardiologist from across town.

The final concern to consider is the cascade of events following a cardiac catheterization. As already noted, there is a risk of significant overestimation of stenosis. Therefore, if a 60 percent blockage in the right coronary artery gets estimated at 70 percent, the medical assessment has been elevated, and the patient goes from being prescribed medication only to now being subjected to stents (or even bypass surgery). Though these stents open the artery and provide a sense of relief that blood flow to the heart is restored, they do nothing to prolong life. There is no difference in the longevity of those who get stents and continue daily use of medication and those who continue daily use of medication without stent placement. The relief of symptoms can be achieved with medication in a large majority of patients.

As you will notice in the upcoming chapters, a stent, when not needed, can lead to considerable harm without any benefit.

What Questions Should I Ask My Doctor if I Am Recommended for Cardiac Catheterization?

- Which of my symptoms are we trying to address with cardiac catheterization?
- Could there be other causes of my symptoms?
- Do I have many risk factors that make blockages more likely?
- Can we perform any noninvasive tests before doing cardiac catheterization?
- (If a stress test has been performed) How bad was my stress test?
- (If your stress test suggests blockages) Can we try medication first, or is it bad enough to perform a heart cath straight away?
- If we find blockages in the coronary artery, am I a candidate for surgery?
- What are my risks from the procedure?

3

Angioplasty: It's Not Killing You!

To the man with only a hammer, every problem looks like a nail.

—Abraham Maslow, paraphrased[1]

ANGIOPLASTY,
AKA PCI,
STENT

Being smart and popular has its perks, but not always . . .

From California to Colorado

Growing up surfing and hiking in California, Saul Dewey realized he was more drawn to the mountains than to the ocean. He made his way to Colorado after graduating from high school, continued to make good grades through college, and got accepted into medical school. An avid hiker and rock climber, Saul found Colorado suited him like a glove. After graduating medical school, he continued his training in orthopedics out there and later settled down in Mountain View, a small Colorado town true to its name. He enjoyed taking care of patients who shared his interest in the outdoors and watching them get back to enjoying life. Running into his previous patients on hiking trails was very gratifying and warmed his heart.

Over the past forty years, Saul had gained an impeccable reputation in this town. His bedside manner was flawless, next only to his skilled hands in the operating room. His ability to connect with everyone from the CEO of the hospital to the servers in the cafeteria had won him many friends. Along the way he had raised a family with his high school sweetheart and now wife, Sally. They had two children, one grandson, and, much to Saul's excitement, another grandchild on the way.

He was getting ready to retire in the next few weeks, looking forward to a long-awaited road trip he and Sally had long dreamed of taking. Immediately after his retirement, they planned to cross the country in an RV, hiking and camping along the way. Saul even had a motor-home agency custom design an RV for them. He was a modest man with simple tastes, but this was going to be his biggest toy. God knew he deserved it!

As the day of his retirement grew closer, however, he found himself experiencing a great loss as he realized he would never treat another patient. After having been the town's most beloved orthopedic doctor for so many years, he felt as though he was undergoing an amputation. In the midst of this gloominess, Saul stopped exercising and no longer took his routine hikes on Saturday. He grew too tired to do much of anything outdoors.

A week before his retirement, Saul was in the hospital sorting through a stack of patient files at the nurses' station when he heard a voice call him from behind. "Days from retirement and still busy, Saul?"

Saul turned around, spotting Jack, a cardiologist, on the other side of the desk. "Oh, hi, Jack; didn't see you there. How're you doing?"

"Same old, same old. Working harder day after day," Jack complained.

But Jack seemed relaxed and free to chat, Saul noticed. That was unusual. "On working hard, my friend, I have got a good one for you: How do you hide a five-dollar bill from a cardiologist?" Saul always had a joke to share.

"You got me. How?"

"Tape it to his kids!" Saul burst out laughing.

Jack saw his life reflected in that joke but shrugged and smiled good-naturedly. "How about you? Looking forward to wrapping up at the office?"

"Yes, but it's bittersweet. This has been my life for nearly forty years." Saul moved closer to Jack to have a more private conversation. "I am feeling a little down about it," he admitted.

"I was wondering if something was going on; I haven't seen you at the golf club lately," Jack noted.

"Just don't feel up to it. I seem to be tired all the time," Saul confessed.

"Are you sure it isn't coronary artery disease? Your blood pressure had been high in the past, and at our age—"

As Jack's pager beeped, the two parted ways, but the brief conversation got Saul's wheels churning. Various things were worrying him, including his road trip, being in the wilderness, and the transition to a new insurance plan. The next morning, he called Jack, and they revisited the fatigue and possibility of testing for coronary artery disease.

"While you are still on the group's insurance, go ahead and do it," Jack suggested. "It can't hurt to check it out."

Saul's stress test was set for the next day—a treadmill test with nuclear dye injection.

During the test, Saul was able to walk and jog for thirteen minutes. The technician performing the test was impressed by his exercise capacity, but when Jack called later that evening, there was concern in his voice.

"Saul, I see changes on the nuclear dye images. They are not gravely concerning, but they aren't completely normal either. I think we should go ahead and do a heart cath and make sure there are no blockages. It's better to have a look and make sure than take the risk." Jack's speech sounded well practiced, and he certainly made it sound like a routine procedure. "I want to make sure you're around for many more years so I can continue to kick your butt on the golf course," Jack laughed, before reassuring Saul that everything would turn out fine and there was no need to worry.

Saul decided to go along with Jack's recommendation. He wanted to make sure that everything was fine before heading out for his long road trip.

A Doctor-Patient Story

Jack squeezed Saul into his tight cath-lab schedule the very next day. Although there had been no spots left, he was happy to adjust it to take care of his friend.

The catheterization was performed first thing in the morning. Through the first half of the procedure, everyone in the room was relaxed, joking and laughing, with Billy Joel playing in the background. However, as Jack examined the right-sided heart arteries, he stopped talking. He was intensely focused on the screen where pictures of Saul's arteries were displayed. The music was muted. After several silent, stress-filled minutes, he came over to Saul, wringing his hands.

"Saul, there is a 70 to 80 percent blockage in the right artery. I think we should do an angioplasty."

Saul merely nodded. The medication to keep him comfortable had put him in la-la land, and he wasn't altogether aware of his surroundings. Before undergoing the cath procedure, he had signed the routine consent form for having angioplasty performed following the cath if needed, so that was permission enough.

The staff prepared for the procedure.

Beginnings in Europe

The story of angioplasty weaves through time and continents with its birth in Europe and evolution in America. At the center of this incredible invention is the visionary Andreas Grüntzig.

Andreas was born in Dresden, along the eastern border of Germany, in 1939 to Wilmar, a chemist, and Charlotta, a teacher. Wilmar passed away when Andreas was six years old. A few years later, Charlotta fled with her children to Argentina to escape poverty, though the family soon returned to Germany in pursuit of a better education for Andreas and his siblings. Andreas was a bright student. He attended high school at one of the oldest public schools in Germany, where celebrities like Johann Sebastian Bach had produced their best work. Luckily, Andreas escaped the eastern part of Germany to the west before the Iron Curtain came down, and he was able to continue his medical education in Heidelberg.[2]

After graduation, Andreas trained and excelled in public health. Here as his teacher said, he learned "to give meticulous care to detail; to know the strength and limitations of one's data; to form intuitive judgments and then to test them by cold reason; to allow neither laziness nor impatience to erode the determination to get it right; and in all these activities, to be guided by the human values of compassion, integrity, and humility."[3] This training would come in handy in Andreas's future career.

After completing successful research on risk factors for heart disease, Andreas found himself drawn to the clinical aspects of vascular medicine. He had learned about the diseases of the arteries in the arms and legs initially while studying in Germany and later in Switzerland, at the University of Zurich. He was deeply influenced by the technique of German physician Eberhard Zeitler, who used small tubes—catheters—of increasing size inside the blocked arteries to expand the artery and improve blood flow. Andreas also spent time observing patients before and after this procedure and noted the salubrious effect of the procedure. He now had a new appreciation for the life-changing impact that opening up blood vessels could have on patients.

Impressed by the new methods he had learned, Andreas returned to Zurich to continue his work on arteries of the limbs. One day, during his rounds, a patient was offered complex open-heart surgery to bypass the blockages in his heart arteries. The patient asked if it would be possible to instead "clean" his obstructed arteries, like a plumber cleans pipes. This question greatly intrigued Andreas, and so he began developing his early ideas on opening up heart arteries to treat the blockages, just as he had been doing with other arteries in the body. Although there were many technical challenges to overcome, he believed that solving this problem was his true calling.

Kitchen Table Talk

Andreas started considering different options and techniques for "cleaning" the heart arteries. The first was to place a latex balloon at the tip of a catheter, pass the catheter inside the partially blocked heart artery, and then inflate the balloon. He spent his evenings working with a team at his kitchen table, discussing and improving this technique. After many failed attempts, he realized that he needed a stiff material to make a balloon, since it had to withstand the high pressure it would be under once inflated to open up the blockages in the arteries. He needed additional experts and outside help to make such a balloon but was unable to convince any company to prototype the catheter he envisioned. And so he and his team continued to struggle and improvise on their own.

Andreas was soon introduced to PVC and experimented with its use. After about a year of tinkering, he had managed to design a balloon capable of withstanding the high pressure required to open a blocked artery. This problem now solved, he turned his focus to making catheters small enough to get to the heart arteries and deliver the balloon to the right location. After many failed attempts and continued improvision, he finally succeeded. To prove its impact, he started experimenting on the heart arteries of dogs, successfully performing the first canine coronary artery dilation in September 1975.[4]

He presented his findings the following year at the meeting of the American Heart Association. Unfortunately, many of the senior cardiologists dismissed his ideas as outlandish. Nevertheless, Andreas was able to find solace in the support of a small minority of US–based cardiologists who found his work impressive.[5]

Returning to Zurich, Andreas continued to work toward applying his technique to the human heart. After testing and retesting his tools, he gained confidence in his invention and grew eager to offer it as an alternative to bypass surgery. However, in his zeal to perform the first human coronary angioplasty, he erred in his choice of first subject: it was a complex case in which this first patient suffered completely clogged arteries of the legs and arms. Andreas's catheters could not pass through the blocked arteries en route to the heart.

He soon realized that he would have to patiently wait and carefully select his next subject. On the lookout for the ideal candidate for another attempt, Andreas and his team waited a full year without success; he even traveled to San Francisco in hopes of recruiting a patient there, but the trip was in vain.

Eventually, an ideal candidate showed up in Zurich. The patient was told that he would be the first in the world to undergo the procedure and that if the procedure failed he would need emergency bypass surgery. The man was open to the idea and consented to the procedure.

On September 16, 1977, the procedure was performed.

Andreas later recalled, "The Chief of Cardiology, the cardiac surgeon, and anesthesiologist, along with cardiology and radiology fellows, were in the recording room to observe the procedure. . . . The guiding catheter was placed. . . . After the first balloon deflation, the distal coronary pressure rose nicely . . . Everyone was surprised about the ease of the procedure, and I started to realize that my dreams had come true."[6]

A new era of angioplasty had dawned, and with it the golden age of cardiology!

Angioplasty Moves to America

However, further progress on the procedure was thwarted. The shackles of tradition and deep-rooted beliefs about the treatment of heart disease in Europe constrained the evolution and spread of Andreas's new invention. And so he began looking across the Atlantic to advance the technique. From among several invitations, he decided to move to Emory University in Atlanta to build a team there. Gone were the days when four people tinkered around a kitchen table; now a large community of cardiologists, technicians, and even small corporations were involved in evolving and refining the technique. By 1980, new catheters had been developed that used better material, were of smaller size, and had softer tips that eased entry into the coronary arteries.[7]

Angioplasty developed at a rapid pace through the early 1980s. It was applied in various other settings—such as during active heart attacks and in multiple coronary arteries. Despite the early success of the procedure in opening the artery, reaccumulation of the blockages remained a challenge. In as many as one-third of the patients undergoing angioplasty, the opened-up coronary artery became blocked off once again. The solution to this problem soon became the holy grail of angioplasty. Powerful blood thinners solved some of the complications in the short term, but long-term answers were needed. One such solution was a tiny metallic tubular mesh, called a *stent*, which had been developed in the 1960s for use in the blocked arteries of the arms and legs. In 1987 the first stent was placed in a coronary artery,[8] and over the next two decades stents evolved thanks to further improvement in their material and structure.

Since Andreas performed the first angioplasty in 1977, the procedure has seen steady acceptance by cardiologists all over the world. Though it went through many iterations, Andreas's original method along with the use of a stent still remains the norm for treatment of blockages in the heart arteries today. Currently more than six hundred thousand of these angioplasties are performed in the United States every year.[9]

Turn for the Worse

Back in Mountain View, Colorado, Saul was surrounded by a flurry of activities in preparation for his angioplasty. The nurse got some blood thinners started, while the technician retrieved Jack's preferred stent and balloon. Another technician clicked away rapidly on his keyboard, documenting everything being done. Within minutes, the team was ready to start the procedure. Jack had been trained at the nation's premier program and had performed these procedures for over seventeen years, with thousands under his belt. He enjoyed performing angioplasties and thrived on them. There was something about the unique adrenaline rush that came from working on heart arteries. Sharing before- and after-stent pictures with patients and their loved ones and noticing initial concern and then relief wash over their faces was incredibly satisfying. Jack never tired of it.

The technician gathered all the equipment for Saul's angioplasty, and, once ready, the catheter was handed to Jack, who leaned over his friend. "You may be a bit uncomfortable on this table, Saul, but give us ten minutes, and we'll be done."

Jack proceeded to position the catheter inside the body, his actions almost automatic at this point. He positioned the catheter at the mouth of the right coronary artery next to the blockage and took a picture. He was horrified to see that the 70 to 80 percent blockage now appeared to be 100 percent, and there was no blood flow! He realized that his catheter had pushed a piece of the clot further and worsened the blockage. He looked up at the heart monitor and, as expected, could see the signs of a heart attack.

He turned to Saul to ask if he was in pain, but before he could say a word, the technician called out, "VF, VF, paddles!"—Saul was in full cardiac arrest, and paddles were required to quickly shock his heart out of the life-threatening arrhythmia.

Jack was stunned. Another team was alerted to come over and help with cardiac resuscitation. The nurse used the paddles to shock Saul. After the first shock, Saul's heart gave three normal beats before reverting back to the fatal rhythm. Another cardiologist came in, and together they quickly devised an action plan, divided the roles, and started reviving Saul. After ten minutes, Saul was placed on a ventilator, and several medications were started to keep his heart in normal rhythm. However, he kept reverting to cardiac arrest. Placing a stent was attempted without success, and a heart surgeon was urgently called. Within an hour, Saul was in the operating room, fighting for his life.

Jack was mortified. He cancelled the rest of his appointments for the day and sat behind his closed office door wondering if he should have waited before rushing in to put in the stent. Was Saul's fatigue truly related to his blockage, or was Jack suffering from *confirmation bias?* Was it right to ignore Saul's excellent exercise capacity and the noncritical nature of the blockage and only consider the information that *confirmed* his existing belief?[10] Should Jack have started his friend on medication before jumping to put in a stent?

From Ohio Valedictorian to Maryland Superstar

Through the 1990s and 2000s, the idea that opening up blocked coronary arteries would benefit one and all gripped the world of cardiology. Angioplasty with a stent was the new lifesaver, and it didn't hurt that the procedure was also well remunerated. The possibility of doing well while doing good attracted the brightest physicians to the field. One such cardiologist was Mark Midei.

Mark graduated as his high school valedictorian in 1975. He earned an expedited medical degree in Ohio and went on to train at the world-renowned Johns Hopkins University. His diligence, intellect, and skill for cardiac procedures earned him a great reputation. After graduation, he rejected an academic job to start his private consulting practice, which grew exponentially, with many other cardiologists joining in to make it the largest cardiology group in the region. But among them all, Mark continued to be the most productive and well-reputed partner.[11]

In a new era of angioplasty in which stents were coated with drugs to prevent them from clogging up, Mark became a superstar. He was an early adopter at the cutting edge of his field, and he believed that he was saving many lives with angioplasties and stents. He was also the busiest and most trusted cardiologist in town. There was a running joke among his friends that, in case of chest pain, one should Sharpie on their chest, "Only Mark Midei, please!" before being rushed to the hospital. The volume of Mark's angioplasty procedures grew exponentially with his reputation.

In 2006, of the near fourteen thousand stent-placement procedures in the state of Maryland, he performed about a thousand of them.[12] Abbott Laboratories, the manufacturer of these stents, looked upon him kindly and bestowed him with many personal favors. Mark's enviable procedural volume drew the attention of hospitals, each hoping to benefit from the income his procedures generated. In 2007, one of the regional hospital systems offered a twenty-five-million-dollar merger package to his private practice group if Mark were a part of the merger.[13] The hospital where he was then practicing, St. Joseph Medical Center, was quite aware of the loss they risked suffering were he to jump ship. It would be devastating for them were Mark Midei to perform all his procedures at a competing hospital. And so they were quick to offer their superstar cardiologist a deal that tripled his salary. He would now be making 1.5 million dollars a year, guaranteed!

Too Good to Be True . . .

And so Mark stayed with St. Joseph Medical Center, collapsing the twenty-five million dollar deal and infuriating many in his group. But for Mark, disaster was around the corner.

Between January and April 2008, the Maryland Board of Physicians received anonymous letters claiming that numerous patients were receiving unneeded stents provided by Mark Midei. Around the same time, St. Joseph's started an internal review of his procedures. The hospital that had so aggressively fought to retain him was now questioning his decision-making. A review by outside consultants determined that his decision to implant stents did not meet the standard of care. They observed that where reviewers saw less than 30 percent blockage, Mark had documented more than 90 percent blockages: It appeared that Mark had intentionally bloated the amount of blockage to justify the stent implant. After the scathing review, Mark was suspended from St. Joseph's Hospital in July 2009. The hospital sent letters to 585 of Mark's former patients alerting them that their stents may have been unwarranted. Numerous lawsuits and a federal investigation followed.

St. Joseph's Medical Center did not escape unscathed. Following a federal investigation, the hospital paid 22 million dollars in fines to cover costs Medicare had incurred financing Mark's unnecessary stent placements. In July 2011, the Maryland Board of Physicians revoked Mark's medical license.[14] Multiple lawsuits from patients harmed by Mark's actions cost the hospital 37 million dollars in settlements.[15]

A Lone Wolf or Part of an Epidemic?

Sadly, Mark Midei's case is by no means the only instance of a rogue cardiologist and a collaborating hospital. Over the past decade, the federal government has brought numerous charges against other cardiologists and hospitals for unnecessary stent placement.[16] Federal investigations of stenting practices have taken place across the country and more than eleven hospitals have settled with federal authorities. In Louisiana, Kentucky, and Maryland, cardiologists have served time in federal prisons for unnecessary stent implants. Between 2010 and 2012, over 1,500 patients received letters from hospitals alerting them that their stents may have been unnecessary.[17]

According to David Brown, a prominent cardiology researcher, in *elective* procedures—as opposed to in emergency cases, such as during heart attacks—two out of three stents placed are unnecessary. Multiple assessments over the years have come to similar conclusions.[18] This amounts to two hundred thousand unneeded stent procedures a year in the United States at a cost of about 2.4 billion dollars annually.[19]

There is wide variation in the use of angioplasty across the United States. In some parts of the country, the rate of angioplasty is three times that of other regions.[20] And yet these increased procedures do not benefit the patient: they correlated to neither a decrease in the chance of future heart attacks nor any increase in life span because of these medically unnecessary procedures.[21]

Interestingly, when cardiologists attend national conferences, away from their practices, there is almost a one-third decrease in the number of angioplasties performed. And yet there is no increase in fatalities resulting from this decrease in the procedure. As a matter of fact, some complex patients do not get angioplasties and *die less often* when cardiologists are away at meetings.[22]

In nonemergent situations, medications have been shown to be as effective as stents in a majority of the patients. However, a large proportion of patients get stents as a first resort before appropriate medicines have been tried—like Saul, in our story in this chapter.[23] This is despite the fact that patients who receive stents risk blood clots, strokes, kidney failure, and bleeding from anticlotting medication. They also risk repeat blockages due to the stent itself, with a resulting increased risk of heart attacks and death. FDA reports suggest that angioplasties and stents have been linked to at least 773 deaths in 2012 alone. And that year there were an additional 4,135 nonfatal stent injuries, such as perforated arteries, blood clots, and strokes, severely tarnishing the idea of the universally positive impact of angioplasty.[24]

Who Gets the Blame?

For a single stent procedure, insurance companies reimburse hospitals approximately twenty thousand dollars. The doctor's fee to perform this forty-five-to ninety-minute procedure is about a thousand dollars. These are obviously very lucrative procedures for hospitals and physicians. It's no wonder, then, that the period between 2001 to 2008 saw a 26 percent increase in the number of hospitals offering angioplasty services.[25] These hospitals compete aggressively to attract physicians who can perform these procedures, offering attractive paychecks to lure high-volume cardiologists. The average salary of a cardiologist performing these procedures is over five hundred thousand dollars per year. In addition, the cost of the procedure rooms where these procedures are performed (called *catheterization labs*), the salaries of the nurses and the technicians assisting in these procedures, and the cost of the necessary equipment all adds up. Once hospitals invest these large sums, they expect to generate an even larger revenue stream through a high number of angioplasties.

Hospitals allocate hefty marketing budgets to put the fear of heart disease into the community. Public "educational" lectures are offered to highlight that heart disease is the commonest cause of death. Newspaper articles, billboard advertisements, and newsletter campaigns reinforce the notion that getting tested and treated for any and all heart conditions is the only way to mitigate the risk of heart-related deaths. Physicians performing a high volume of procedures are rewarded through large bonuses, and the highest-performing physicians are rewarded through administrative positions with high salaries and very few responsibilities. All of these factors combine to create an environment where the science of cardiology and consideration of patient care is lost in the process.

Americans have come to believe the rhetoric: patients worry that any amount of blockage in the heart arteries brings them closer to death by increasing the chance of a fatal heart attack but believe that opening up the artery will prevent this fate.

As we have already discussed here, angioplasty performed in nonemergent situations has not been shown to prolong life by a single day. But according to one report, patients who had given *informed consent* to undergo angioplasty were asked, "How much of an increase in your life span do you expect to get out of this procedure?"

Their typical answer? Ten years![26]

After being informed that angioplasty would *not* prevent future heart attacks, two out of five of these patients continued to believe that it would. Half of the patients continued to choose angioplasty despite recognizing the lack of benefit and the risk of the procedure. It is clear that it is hard to reverse long-held belief that any amount of blockage in the heart is the kiss of death.[27]

Research suggests that over 50 percent of cardiologists either implicitly or explicitly overstate the benefits of angioplasty. Even a proven understanding of the lack of benefit did not change the bloating of these benefits to the patient. Indeed, the cardiologists held fast to this misunderstanding even when they had no financial incentive to recommend the procedure.[28] There may be an element of *belief bias*, or a tendency to persevere in one's belief even when research shows the fallacy in it.[29] This is a cognitive error, or an error in the physician's way of thinking. Physicians have been convinced that having unimpeded blood flow through open heart arteries is necessary for normal life.[30] By extension, physicians believe that any blockage in the heart artery is life-threatening and that opening up the blocked artery reverses this hazard. The satisfaction one derives from seeing the before and after pictures of the blocked artery seemingly overwhelm any recognition of the lack of benefit to the patient. Time and time again, research studies have shown that, heart attacks aside, opening the heart artery does not increase life span.[31] However, cardiologists persist in their belief to the contrary, despite clear and indisputable evidence otherwise, whether because of personal conviction or financial motivation.

It is well understood that financial incentive does have its perils: patients who have private insurance with high levels of reimbursement tend to get inappropriate procedures at twice the rate that uninsured patients do.[32] Higher patient expectations, belief bias, and financial rewards lead to increased procedures regardless of true medical necessity.[33]

Not an Appropriate Send-Off

Saul's surgery lasted four hours, and he came out of it with a normal heart rhythm and cleared blockages. Unfortunately, the multiple episodes of cardiac arrest had deprived his brain and heart of vital blood supply for long periods. Over the next twenty-four hours, several medications were tried to keep his blood pressure under control, but he kept going into cardiac arrest. Eventually, his family realized that further intervention would be futile. Even if he were to make it by some miracle, he would be in a permanent vegetative state, no longer able to kiss his wife or take his beloved hikes. That was not what Saul would have wanted for himself. After grave discussion and many tears, the family decided to withdraw support and let him go with peace and dignity. Saul passed away on the day of his retirement.

APPENDIX

What Are Coronary Arteries?

As discussed in chapter 2, *coronary arteries* supply blood to the heart. The heart gets its own blood supply from two major blood vessels—the left main artery and the right coronary artery. The left main artery divides further into two branches. These two branches along with the right coronary artery form the three major arteries supplying blood to the heart (see figure 3.1).

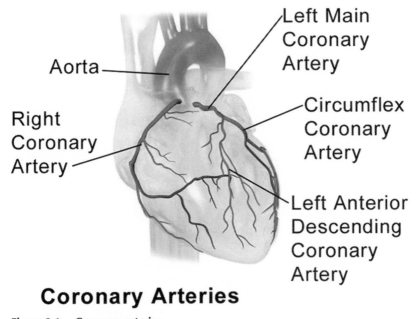

Coronary Arteries

Figure 3.1.   Coronary arteries
Blausen Medical Communication, Inc.

As we age, plaque is deposited in the arteries. This creates blockage in the blood flow to the heart muscles. The process happens gradually over an individual's lifetime, but factors such as smoking, diabetes, high blood pressure, high cholesterol, and a family history of blockages in these arteries before the age of fifty-five can increase the rate of plaque buildup (see figure 3.2).

Although good blood flow through these arteries is essential to keeping the heart muscle healthy and functioning, it can continue to function normally even with 50 to 60 percent blockage (except in the left main artery, where anything more than 50 percent blockage is concerning).

When there is a 70 percent blockage in the artery, it is considered significant enough to act on. Coronary arteries that have less than 70 percent blockage do not need intervention by stents or bypass surgery; the only exception, as noted previously, is the left main artery, where a 50 percent blockage gives sufficient cause for concern. There is no benefit from the placement of stents or bypass surgery in coronary arteries that are blocked less than 70 percent.[34] Although it may sound scary when your doctor says you have a 60 percent blockage, do not sign up to do something that may hurt you more than the blockage itself.

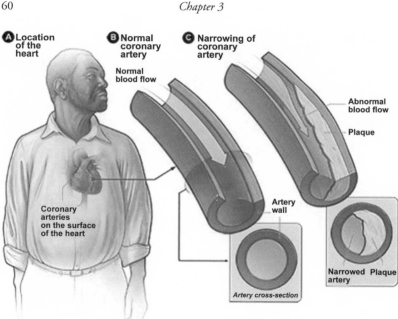

Figure 3.2.   Coronary artery disease
National Institutes of Health

People live a perfectly normal life at 60 percent blockage without requiring stents or bypass surgery.

As mentioned, these blockages build up gradually over a period of time. So, when your doctor says that a 90 percent blockage has been found, it is important to remember that you have likely lived with the same degree of blockage for weeks, if not months. Therefore, do not rush into a decision or fear that if you do not take care of it right away any delay will be catastrophic. You lived with the same degree of blockage yesterday, the day before, and perhaps weeks before that. There is also ample research to show that these 90 percent blockages rarely cause heart attacks and that heart attacks are never the result of mature 70, 80, 90, or even 95 percent blockages.

What Is Angioplasty? What Is a Stent?

Angioplasty is the procedure used to open up the blocked coronary arteries and enable normal blood flow to the heart muscle. It is performed by threading a catheter through a puncture in the leg or arm artery to the coronary

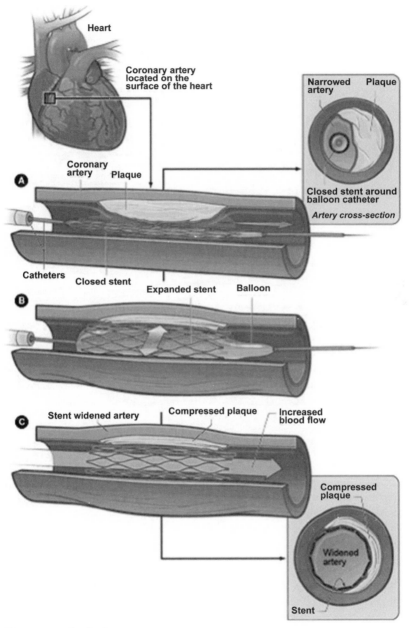

Heart

Coronary artery located on the surface of the heart

Narrowed artery **Plaque**

Closed stent around balloon catheter

Artery cross-section

A

Coronary artery **Plaque**

Catheters **Closed stent**

B

Expanded stent **Balloon**

C

Stent widened artery **Compressed plaque** **Increased blood flow**

Compressed plaque

Widened artery

Stent

Figure 3.3. Angioplasty
National Institutes of Health

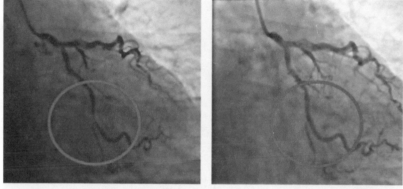

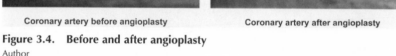

Coronary artery before angioplasty   Coronary artery after angioplasty

Figure 3.4.   Before and after angioplasty
Author

arteries. A small balloon is inflated within the blocked artery to push the plaque toward the wall of the artery and thus clear the path for blood flow. Angioplasty is very often combined with the placement of a small wire mesh tube, called a *stent*, to help prop the artery open and decrease its chance of narrowing again (see figures 3.3 and 3.4).

When performed under the *emergent* circumstances of a heart attack with ongoing active chest pain, shortness of breath, or other symptoms and the artery is 100 percent blocked, opening these arteries and restoring the blood flow will be tremendously helpful and ultimately save your life.

However, when performed under *elective* circumstances with 70, 80, 90, or even 95 percent blockage, angioplasty will not increase your life span or prevent future major heart attacks. It will help any symptoms you may have that are related to these blockages, such as chest pain, shortness of breath, increased fatigue, and so on, though the same benefit may be derived from taking medication, which would prevent invasive procedures.

Under elective circumstances with a 95 percent blockage, elective angioplasty will not prevent your next major heart attack or prolong your life.[35]

I was told that if my 90 percent blockage becomes 100 percent I can have a heart attack. So, I need a stent to open up this blockage. So, this stent will prevent a heart attack right?

A heart attack is caused by 100 percent blockage in one of the coronary arteries. Such a complete blockage is caused by a blood clot in the coronary artery.

Patients with coronary artery disease have plaques of fat, cholesterol, etc. covered with a thin lining of fibrinous matter. These plaques could be minor and causing as little as a 30 percent blockage. If this thin lining covering the plaque is damaged, a rapid reaction takes place and within hours a blood clot forms on top of this minor plaque. Such a blood clot causes a complete blockage of the coronary artery and cuts off the blood supply completely. This leads to a heart attack, also called myocardial infarction. If this is not treated immediately, the heart muscle which was dependent on that artery for blood supply is damaged.

The lining on the 90 percent blockage is mature and unlikely to be damaged and form clot on top of it. So, it is not the 90 percent blockage which has built up over weeks, months and years which goes on to develop the 100 percent block and heart attack. Instead, the sudden formation of a blood clot on top of a minor plaque with its thin, immature lining is responsible for heart attack.

When is an Angioplasty or a Stent Needed?

If you are having a heart attack with ongoing chest pain or shortness of breath and an EKG indicating heart attack, an emergency angioplasty will save your life.

In the case of *elective* procedures, patients with one or more coronary arteries (other than the left main artery) blocked more than 70 percent who continue to have symptoms such as those described above because of low blood flow to the heart muscle despite treatment with medication and lifestyle modification may be candidates for angioplasty and stent placement. An angioplasty performed under these circumstances combined with ongoing medication use will help decrease symptoms.

If the left main artery is blocked more than 50 percent, bypass surgery is preferred. Under rare circumstances an angioplasty may be performed instead.

Angioplasty is not generally needed or recommended for blockages less than 70 percent. For such blockages, lifestyle changes and medication are appropriate treatment options. If you have no symptoms, there is no benefit to having an angioplasty or a stent. It is neither going to reduce the chance of a future heart attack nor increase your life span.[36]

What Are the Risks of Angioplasty?

Like any invasive procedure, there are risks to angioplasty. Careful consideration of the potential complications will help you assess whether the benefit of the procedure is worth the risks. Elective procedures are exactly that—*elective*. Since your life is not in imminent danger, there is adequate time to think about and make a decision regarding the procedure.

Here are some of the risks of angioplasty and stent procedures:

- Bleeding at the site where the tiny tube was inserted
- Damage to the blood vessel where the tiny tube was inserted
- Possible sudden closure of the coronary artery leading to a heart attack (Not only does angioplasty not prevent heart attacks, it may *cause* them as a complication of the procedure.)
- A small tear in the inner lining of the coronary artery and the need for more angioplasty than previously planned
- Increased risk of needing urgent bypass surgery
- Renarrowing of the coronary artery that was opened (restenosis), requiring repeat angioplasty
- Kidney problems resulting from the dye used in the procedure
- Increased potential for a stroke due to clots breaking up during the procedure and blocking off the blood vessels supplying the brain
- Possibility of death as a result of the procedure, which is higher when more than one artery is involved or the patient has other high-risk medical conditions[37]

What Questions Should I Ask My Cardiologist before Signing Up for a Stent Procedure?

Start by asking your cardiologist to explain the evidence from your testing that suggests you need an angioplasty. Ask your doctor,

- Which arteries are blocked?
- What percent of those arteries are blocked?
- Do you believe this is elective or emergent angioplasty?
- Can we try medication to address my symptoms first?
- Will I have increased life span with angioplasty or with bypass surgery for these blockages?
- What are the risks of the procedure? Am I in the high-risk category?
- Will this procedure help me feel better?
- Will this procedure help me live longer? By how many months/years?

4

Bypass Surgery:
A Second Opinion

Fools rush in where angels fear to tread.

—Alexander Pope[1]

BYPASS SURGERY
AKA CORONARY ARTERY BYPASS GRAFTING
OR CABG (PRONOUNCED "CABBAGE")

A Ticking Time Bomb?

But I've been feeling so good, Richard wondered. *How can this be?*

Losing his fifty-five-year-old father to heart attack had been a shock to Richard. Becoming the oldest in their family at the age of twenty-eight, he felt responsible for his younger siblings. He realized that he was their role model and so turned his life around. He began focusing on his work and building his career, stopped smoking, and started exercising. Over time, he was able to convince his younger siblings to adopt equally healthy lifestyles to avoid meeting their father's fate.

Now at sixty-two years of age, Richard looked younger than his peers. He played singles tennis three days a week and easily kept up with the players in his league. He believed that annual checkups with his cardiologist, Dr. Nohi, were ensuring that he had a healthy heart, so he had diligently kept his appointment every year.

As he had at every checkup, Dr. Nohi recommended a stress test this year. Over the years, Richard had gotten competitive with his stress test and used his treadmill time to benchmark his health. This year, he was very happy he was able to run on the treadmill for over twelve minutes and was expecting the nurse's routine call of "All looks good, Richard!"

To his surprise, the day after the test, Dr. Nohi called him at home. "Richard, the heart pumping looks normal, but I saw a problem on the EKG around the twelve-minute mark of the stress test. We'd better schedule a cardiac catheterization."

Dr. Nohi went on to explain that catheterization was a procedure in which a small tube was inserted into the heart arteries and dye was injected into them. He was confident, he told Richard, that this was the best way to tell if there were blockages in the heart arteries. It was a routine procedure, he assured Richard, and it was always "better to be safe than sorry."

The turn of events left Richard puzzled. Physically, he had been feeling great. Nevertheless, he trusted Dr. Nohi and consoled himself that it never hurt to look. He felt uncomfortable with the procedure but would not put his health on the line.

*   *   *

Richard followed the instructions Dr. Nohi had given him, not eating or drinking anything after midnight the day before the procedure. He showed up at the hospital on the assigned day, surprised to see that the place seemed like a factory. He was quickly informed that he was fifth in line. His hopes for an early lunch disappeared, as after severe delays his 10 o'clock time slot kept being pushed back, and finally at 2 p.m. he was taken in for the procedure. The medication he received made him sleep through it, and he woke up in the recovery area.

He waited for news until 5 p.m., when Dr. Nohi came back to tell him what he had found out. Shockingly, Dr. Nohi opened with, "Richard, we'll admit you tonight, and you'll be seen by a surgeon in the morning. You need bypass surgery. I am glad we caught this in time; it's dangerous enough that we cannot let you go home."

The doctor went on to describe the details of the blockages and procedure, but Richard was too depressed to focus on what was being said. He just could not make sense of this situation.

But I've been feeling so good. How can this be? Will I meet my father's fate? Should I make a will before the surgery? Do I have time? Should I call my siblings and let them know? How will they react to this?

After a sleepless night, Richard got ready to meet his surgeon the next morning. The nurses told him that this was the busiest and most well-reputed surgeon in town and that Richard shouldn't have any concerns.

When the surgeon arrived, he got straight down to business. "Dr. Nohi says you need bypass surgery. I've gone over your chart, and I'm not worried; it'll be straightforward, and you'll be out of here in four to five days. We have the surgery scheduled, but I have two emergency cases today, so we'll have to do it tomorrow. Alright?"

Before Richard could even nod, his surgeon was out the door.

Germany's Conquest of Europe and CABG's Conquest of Heart Disease

What happened to Richard occurs every day in hundreds of hospitals across the United States: It starts with an annual physical, or "routine" stress test, where a spot found here or there on a scan or a minor blip on the EKG is quickly followed by a cardiac catheterization and then a stent or bypass surgery. The whole process is overwhelmed by a feeling of "Thank God we looked!" along with a sense that the patient had been sitting on a ticking time bomb.

The story of *coronary artery bypass grafting*—or *CABG* surgery, as it is known—begins almost a century ago, when treatment for blocked arteries still stymied medicine's quest to conquer heart disease. In the 1920s, autopsy findings documented the presence of blockages in the heart arteries—or coronary arteries—among patients with chest pain. It was recognized that these blockages were the cause of low blood flow to the heart muscle. Lack of blood flow and oxygen to the heart muscle were recognized as causes of chest pain and, in some cases, death.[2] In the 1930s in order to get blood supply to the heart muscle, surgeons attached small pieces of muscle along with blood supply. They hoped that the blood supply from the muscle would help the heart muscle next to it. However, this method failed and did little to benefit the patients. In the 1940s, attention turned to one of the arteries that traversed close to the heart and supplied blood to the chest wall and the breast. Various attempts were made to reposition this artery on the heart muscle to provide enough oxygen directly to the heart, but these attempts also fell short. It was soon postulated that the only way to provide blood supply to the heart muscle affected by the blocked artery would be to connect the end of another artery directly to the blocked one at a location beyond the blockage. This would create a *bypass* of the blockage, so to speak, but was going to be technically difficult. It would require an especially gifted mind to overcome the many challenges and succeed at this task.

Vasilii Kolesov was born in 1904 in a small village in Russia's northwest. The son of well-to-do farmers, Vasilii went to Leningrad to study medicine. Upon graduation, he was ordered to work as a physician in a metallurgical factory.

This did not quench his desire to improve, innovate, or excel, and he soon he returned to Leningrad for further surgical study. Upon completing this training, he became an academic surgeon at the Institute of Post-Graduate Medical Studies. However, World War II soon interrupted his career, and he was commanded to be surgeon-in-chief in one of Leningrad's municipal hospitals.

For almost two and a half years, German troops surrounded the city, cutting its residents off from the rest of Russia and the world. Along with the resilient people of Leningrad, Vasilii endured great physical and mental hardship, but he managed to continue his work through Nazi bombardment and widespread famine. In one particularly harrowing incident, a bomb exploded directly outside the facility where Vasilii was performing surgery. A piece of shell ricocheted to the ceiling, sending dust and dirt cascading down toward the open surgical wound, when Vasilii leaned over to shield his patient with his own body.

In the winter of 1942, midway through the longest and most destructive siege in human history, the bitter cold and lack of food led to thousands of deaths throughout the city.[3] The Kolesov family was not immune; several of Vasilii's relatives died, and Vasilii himself briefly endured a potentially fatal inflammation of the heart at only thirty-eight years of age. But he managed to recover completely and was soon able to return to the service of his country.

At the close of January 1944, the long Siege of Leningrad finally ended when Soviet troops managed to expel Nazi invaders from the city. Vasilii hoped this would mean the return of some semblance of normalcy in which he could resume his academic career. But instead he was called upon to join the medical corps and follow the Red Army's advance into Poland.

Fate intervened at the very last moment, however: As Vasilii boarded the train to the front, he was recalled by his superiors to join the new Department of Cardiovascular Surgery at the Military Medical Academy. And it was here that Vasilii Kolesov started his path to heart surgery.

As he continued his work, he soon became chief of surgery at the First Leningrad Medical Institute. Here he conducted several cardiac-surgery experiments on dogs, refining techniques that would later be introduced worldwide and come to define the procedure: He had previously read about a CABG surgery performed on a patient by a team of surgeons at the Albert Einstein College of Medicine and decided to try to replicate the results in dogs. During these canine surgeries Vasilii made certain critical revisions to the procedure: He devised special instruments that allowed him to suture blood vessels to one another. He further modified other surgical equipment as well as magnifying glasses that made the delicate surgery possible. He was now able to connect

small arteries to one another and fine-tune various other aspects of the procedure. After performing successful surgery on a total of eight dogs over a
nineteen-month period, he undertook surgery on a human patient.

On February 25, 1964, at not quite sixty years of age, using the skill and
expertise he had slowly built up over his lifetime, Vasilii Kolesov successfully
connected a nearby artery to a location beyond the blockage in a patient's
coronary artery—a procedure that had been postulated more than two decades ago. Vasilii's refined techniques revolutionized coronary artery bypass
grafting, making it one of the most-performed procedures in the quest to
defeat heart disease.[4] He had performed surgeries through the Nazi bomb-
ing of Leningrad, nearly died of heart disease himself, and narrowly avoided
being sent off to the Red Army Medical Corps in Poland where fighting was
intense. And now he was responsible for the dawn of a new era in CABG
surgery. The world's quarter-century wait for bypass surgery was finally over.

Marching On

Over the years, the technique of coronary artery bypass grafting continued
to be refined and fine-tuned. But despite Vasilii's brilliance, there remained one
major hurdle: the blocked coronary arteries eligible for bypass were still limited
by the number of alternative arteries present in the vicinity of the heart.

In 1967 an Argentine surgeon working at the Cleveland Clinic used redun-
dant leg veins to bypass blocked coronary arteries, eliminating this concern
once and for all. René Favaloro used small pieces of a single leg vein to connect to his patient's aorta—the largest artery in the chest—beyond the blocked
artery, enabling René to bypass multiple blocked arteries. Due to his surgical
skill and the tremendous need for the procedure, by the end of that year René
had performed it on 180 patients. The technique continued to be mastered
over the coming years, and this once-curious procedure gained acceptance
by the mainstream medical community.[5] This led to a rapid increase in the
number of procedures performed. The annual number of CABG procedures
in the United States increased from about thirty thousand in 1974 to half a
million in 2012.[6]

We Can Do It, but Does It Help?

Once CABG surgery became more refined and routine, surgeons believed
that its impact was self-evident: The heart muscle requires oxygen to be delivered through the coronary arteries, and when the blockage of coronary arteries

by plaque prevents oxygen from getting there, the bypass grafts get around the blockage, thereby providing the much-needed oxygen. That was the end of the story, as far as they were concerned.

However, by the last quarter of the twentieth century, cardiologists—their nonsurgical colleagues—began questioning the efficacy of CABG over medication and wanted to address the issue in clinical trials.[7] The initial studies, which included only a few patients, did not show any improvement in terms of longevity or the prevention of future heart attacks in those undergoing CABG compared to those taking medication only. However, those undergoing CABG did show improved symptoms including chest pain compared to those on medication alone.

When the studies were later reassessed with a much larger group of patients combined from various studies, an improvement in longevity was evident among those undergoing CABG. Over the ten-year period after initial evaluation, 30 percent of the patients receiving medication died, compared to only 26 percent of those who had undergone CABG. There were patient groups with specific patterns of blockages that benefitted a lot more from CABG, gaining an increased life span as well as a symptom-free life.[8]

An Escape to Safety

After the surgeon swept out of the room, Richard was left reeling: in the span of a few days he'd gone from a routine stress test to prepping for open-heart surgery. He made a phone call to his physician friend, Ron, who was in his tennis league, recounting the story of what had happened and sharing his disbelief that even though he felt so healthy he was being told he needed this emergency surgery.

"All this is happening so suddenly. I just wish I had made a will. I don't know if I should let my brother and sister know. This is all happening very fast, but I guess if this saves my life, I don't have much of a choice, do I?"

"You didn't have a heart attack recently, did you?"

"No, it was a routine stress test. I walked in yesterday morning for this elective procedure, and now I need surgery," Richard explained.

"Did they tell you if your heart pumping is low?"

Ron seemed to be looking for reasons for the urgency of the surgery, and Richard suddenly felt glad he had made contact. "No, my heart has been pumping normally. I remember Dr. Nohi telling me that."

Ron sighed. "Listen, my friend. If you trust me, request a discharge for now. Let's get a second opinion."

Richard liked the sound of that; time for a second opinion meant less urgency than he had thought, but something still bothered him. "Ron, I trust you completely, but you know that Dr. Nohi has an excellent reputation. He is the busiest cardiologist in town, and this surgeon is also second to none around here."

Ron hummed, understanding his friend's fear, but remaining skeptical. "Well, I'll arrange a second opinion for you in a week if you want. I think that CABG tomorrow would be rushing into things, and I don't understand the need to hurry. Even if you do need the surgery, I truly believe we can wait a week." He paused to let his words sink in, then reaffirming, "I would get a discharge from the hospital to seek that second opinion if I were you."

Richard did not need any more convincing. As per Ron's suggestion, he requested a discharge and a copy of his cardiac catheterization results. But he was confused about the variation in opinion: here were Dr. Nohi and his team asking him to get CABG surgery, and another physician had confidently asked him to get discharged in order to reexamine the cardiac catheterization results! However, if there was even a 5 percent chance of avoiding surgery without taking a chance on his life, Richard was all for it.

* * *

In the days that followed, while Richard scurried around seeking a lawyer and making his will, Ron pulled some strings and got an appointment for Richard with Dr. Bailey, a cardiologist at the university hospital. Richard noted how different this visit was: He was asked lots of questions about his overall health, his activities, and the details of his medical history. Even after looking at the cardiac catheterization film, Dr. Bailey seemed to focus more on various aspects of Richard's medical history—something neither Dr. Nohi nor the cardiac surgeon had paid much attention to.

"Let me be very sure of what you are saying," the doctor said to Richard. "You do not have chest pain or pressure, no shortness of breath, no jaw pain—just a little fatigue. You were also on the treadmill for twelve minutes during the stress test. Is that right?"

Richard nodded.

"Well, CABG helps in resolution of symptoms for those who continue to have them even *after* they have been tried on medication. It can also result in an increased life span in a very select group of patients."

"But I don't feel any different; I don't have any symptoms," Richard insisted.

Dr. Bailey smiled. "Yes. The only role of surgery will be to increase your life span, and that's only if you belong to a group of patients with a specific disease pattern."

"Do I have that disease pattern on the cardiac catheterization?" Richard asked quickly. The answer could not come fast enough.

"As per guidelines from the American College of Cardiology, you get the benefit of improved survival *if*"—Bailey ticked the categories off on his fingers—"you have blockage in the main coronary artery on the left side, *which you do not*; you have blockages in all three coronary arteries, *which you do not*; or you have low pumping function in addition to blockages in the heart, *which you do not*." The doctor sat back in his chair. "I do not believe that your life is in jeopardy from the blockages here. Therefore, doing CABG surgery for these blockages will not increase your longevity, since it's not under siege anyway."

"So I don't need surgery?" Richard clarified.

"Correct. There is no need for CABG in your case," Dr. Bailey concluded.

"So why did Dr. Nohi and the cardiac surgeon recommend CABG for me?" Richard could not hold back his question.

Dr. Bailey merely smiled.

When the Going Gets Good . . .

The smile was neither satisfying nor reassuring for Richard. Dr. Bailey had made recommendations for possible lifestyle changes and medication, and Richard headed back home, where he fired up his laptop and Googled "unnecessary CABG" and "unneeded bypass surgery."

Among the various results appearing on the screen, Richard was particularly shocked to read the case of Redding Medical Center in Redding, California. This 238–bed hospital had been touted as the best in a town of eighty thousand people, mostly due to the high volume of cardiac procedures undertaken there. Cardiologist Chae Hyun Moon and cardiac surgeon Fidel Realyvasquez had been the rock stars of the center. The hospital had gone to great lengths to support these doctors, who were looked upon as rainmakers. The administration had built a cardiac center to support their practice, and it yielded great results.

Redding Medical Center's annual income doubled during the five-year period from 1998 to 2002 to a high of ninety-four million dollars—twenty times higher than the income at the competing hospital in town. After being treated at the hospital, many patients would talk about being advised to let the cardiac team have a look at their coronary arteries. Some claimed that these doctors had saved their lives, but others spoke of the pressure they felt they'd been subjected to, having been told, "If you don't sign up for this procedure, you are going to die."

Dr. Moon recommended emergency CABG surgery to many of his patients, which was usually performed by Dr. Realyvasquez, the hospital's cardiac surgeon. Redding Medical Center soon led California in the number of CABG surgeries performed. Over the years, some local physicians, technicians, and nursing staff, as well as patients themselves, brought up concerns regarding the overuse of these cardiac surgeries at the hospital. However, no internal evaluation was conducted to validate or refute these complaints. The cash flow was powerful enough for administrators to not only ignore the concerns but also reward the two physicians running the program with positions on hospital boards and roles as directors.[9]

When Father John Corapi, a Catholic priest living in the Redding area, made an appointment with Dr. Moon to discuss his heart health, he had an experience that a lot of Redding patients would have found familiar. Father Corapi was advised to undergo the CABG procedure for his "fatal" heart condition. Trusting this recommendation, he made his will and went to another hospital for his CABG procedure, because some of his friends worked there.[10] To his surprise, the cardiologist there looked at the angiography of the coronary arteries (cardiac cath) performed at Redding Medical Center and came to a conclusion that surgery was not needed. Father Corapi was puzzled by this difference in opinion and sought opinions from several other cardiologists. They all confirmed that he did not need bypass surgery or indeed any other procedures. When Father Corapi brought this to the attention of the administrators at Redding Medical Center, they did not heed his complaint. After several phone calls all the way up to the CEO fell on deaf ears, Father Corapi called the FBI.

Based on his account, along with other complaints they'd received, in the fall of 2002 federal agents raided Redding Medical Center and confiscated documents pertaining to these surgeries.[11] These files contained the records of 167 patients who had died after undergoing surgery recommended by Dr. Moon. As per the affidavit by the FBI, up to 50 percent of the procedures that the cardiologist and the cardiac surgeon had performed at Redding Medical Center may not have been necessary.[12] The affidavit also asserted that the cardiologist performed four to five times as many cardiac catheterization procedures as his peers in California.

Following this disclosure, a total of 769 people sued the hospital and the doctors, claiming they had been operated on unnecessarily. As a result, the doctors' malpractice insurance companies and Redding Medical Center's parent company, Tenet Healthcare Corporation, paid out more than half a billion dollars in compensation. Both of the physicians involved in the scandal also lost their licenses to practice medicine.[13]

Richard closed his laptop soberly, disturbed by what he had read.

A Perfect Storm

Why does unnecessary surgery happen? To satisfy doctors' greed? To provide hope? To increase hospital profits?

We believe that perfect functioning of the heart is critical to survival, and more widely it is believed that anything out of place, however minor, needs to be fixed. Even when physicians make no mention of it, patients take it as "obvious" that if there is anything wrong with their heart it needs to be fixed, or else death is imminent. In some cases, this may be true, but in a large majority of cases patients take the leap of creating a catastrophe in their mind even when the issue is minor.

Once such a fear of impending disaster has taken hold, the patient assumes that the issue needs to be fixed and that the more invasive the procedure is the more beneficial it is and the better off the patient will be.[14] It is an article of faith that if the surgeon puts hours into the procedure and it takes place right away, then the procedure has to be beneficial and lifesaving. We have gradually come to believe that having these procedures is better than inaction. Therefore, we also believe that these procedures and surgeries are exclusively an act of prolonging or saving lives—at least until we are told otherwise.

These unrealistic expectations have made patients more eager to have procedures. Physicians themselves favor these procedures—even when reasonable, equally effective, and in many cases *safer* treatment options involving medication are available.[15] The extraordinary rate of remuneration that surgeries and procedures attract in the fee-for-service model of health care adds more fuel to the fire.

A scared patient looking to a trusted but well-incentivized physician for a quick surgical fix creates the potential for overuse of surgeries and procedures. As in Richard's story, and in the case of those patients in Redding, it is amazing how the fear of death can motivate patients to agree to anything the doctor suggests, even if there is scientific evidence against the procedure the doctor suggests. Though in the right patient CABG is helpful, in the wrong patient it is a reckless procedure. The risk of death to some heart patients while on the right medication may be so small that the surgical risk of CABG surgery is not worthwhile.

There is wide variation nationwide in the number of CABG surgeries performed. Certain regions of the country have five times as many CABG surgeries performed as others, yet there is no regional difference in number of heart-disease related deaths.[16] Compared to their Canadian peers, patients in the United States underwent CABG procedures 7.5 times more often after a heart attack. However, they lived no longer, had no fewer heart attacks, and presented no fewer symptoms than did the Canadian patients.[17]

The patient expectation of action in the form of "lifesaving procedures," the cardiologists' and cardiac surgeons' own desire to "act" to save their patient's life, and the perverse incentive of the fee-for-service model has created the perfect storm in the United States. That said, it is the fee-for-service system and the attitudes it breeds that is accountable for such high rates of unnecessary bypass surgery. Doctors are not bad, but the system can make them so. If you pay more for procedures, you get more procedures, whether they are cardiac catheterizations, stents, or CABGs.

As such, increasing numbers of hospitals have rapidly created surgical programs to offer CABG surgeries, knowing they will profit considerably. Over the past few years, CABG procedures have shifted from being performed in high-volume academic centers and regional medical centers to being performed in low-volume community hospitals. Unfortunately, this has also increased the risk to patients. The risk of procedures at low-volume centers that perform fewer than 150 CABG procedures a year is greater than the risk at locations with a higher volume of procedures. It is estimated that this shift has probably resulted in 190 additional deaths in 2003 alone.[18]

Happily Ever After

Richard was jarred by what he'd read about unnecessary CABG. Armed with this understanding and the lifestyle recommendations Dr. Bailey had made for him, Richard diligently focused on living a healthier life: He improved his diet, continued to exercise on a regular basis, and was consistent in his use of prescribed medication.

Seven years passed since the whole ordeal, and over time Richard began advising many of his friends and colleagues on the importance of getting a second opinion and exploring nonsurgical options before undergoing an "emergency" surgery as a result of a routine stress test or cardiac catheterization.

He felt that he had been saved from the physical trauma and mental agony of a CABG surgery he had never needed.

APPENDIX

What Are Coronary Arteries?

As we've seen previously, *coronary arteries* supply blood to the heart muscle. The heart gets its own blood supply from two major blood vessels—the left main artery and right coronary artery. The left main artery divides further into two branches. These branches, along with the right coronary artery, form the three major arteries supplying blood to the heart (see figure 4.1).

As we age, plaque is deposited in the arteries. This creates blockages for the blood flow to the heart muscles—or coronary artery disease (see figure 4.2). Factors such as smoking, diabetes, high blood pressure, high cholesterol, or a family history of blockages in these arteries before the age of fifty-five can increase the rate of plaque buildup. Although good blood flow through these arteries is essential to keeping the heart muscle healthy and functioning at its best, the heart muscle can continue to function normally even with a 50 to 60 percent blockage (except in the left main artery, where anything more than 50 percent blockage is concerning).

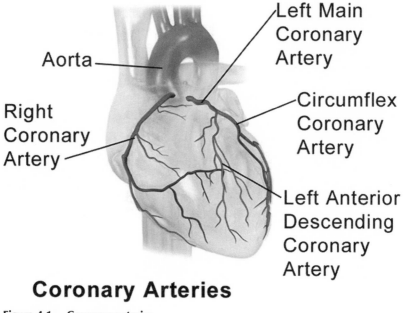

Figure 4.1.   Coronary arteries
Blausen Medical Communication, Inc.

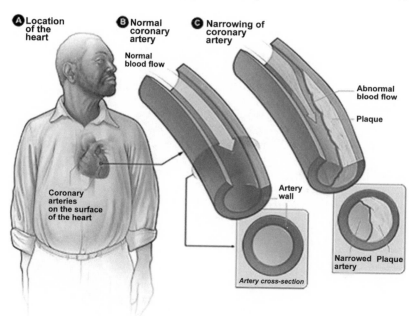

Figure 4.2.   Coronary artery disease
National Institutes of Health

When there is a 70 percent blockage in the artery, it is considered to be a significant enough blockage to act on. Coronary arteries that have less than 70 percent blockage do not need intervention by stents or CABG surgery; the only exception, as noted earlier, is the left main artery, where 50 percent blockage is enough to be of concern. There is no benefit from the placement of stents or doing CABG surgery on coronary arteries that are blocked less than 70 percent. Although it may sound scary when your doctor says you have a 60 percent blockage, do not sign up to do something that may hurt you more than the blockage itself. People live a perfectly healthy and normal life at 60 percent blockage without requiring stents or bypass surgery.[19] (See figures 4.3 and 4.4.)

What Is CABG, or Bypass Surgery?

CABG is one treatment for blockages in the coronary arteries. During CABG, a healthy artery or vein from the body is connected, or grafted, to a blocked coronary artery. The grafted artery or vein *bypasses*—goes around—the blocked portion of the coronary artery. This creates a new path for oxygen-rich

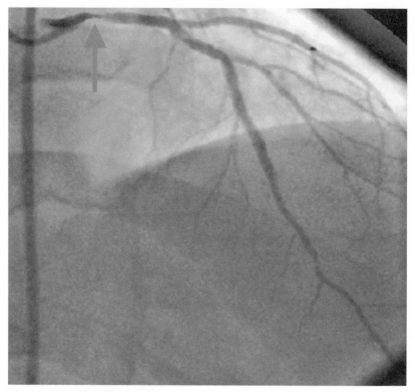

Figure 4.3.   Left main disease
Muhammad Shammin Siddiqui

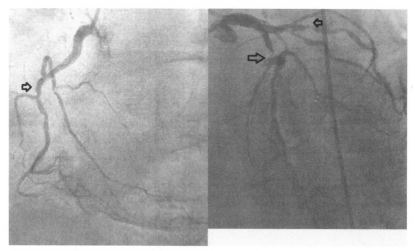

Figure 4.4.   Three vessel disease
Author

blood to flow to the heart muscle. During a single CABG procedure, multiple blockages in the coronary arteries can be bypassed (see figure 4.5).

When Does a Patient Need CABG?

Here is what the American College of Cardiology and American Heart Association recommend in terms of CABG surgery:

- CABG is recommended ***to increase life span*** in patients (even if they have no symptoms)
  - There is more than 50 percent blockage in left main artery
  - There is more than 70 percent blockage in all three coronary arteries
  - There is more than 70 percent blockage in the early portion of the left anterior descending artery *and* one more artery
  - There is more than 70 percent blockage in two coronary arteries *and* a very abnormal stress test
  - There is more than 70 percent blockage in two coronary arteries *and* heart-pumping function between 35 to 50 percent (normal is 55 to 65 percent).[20]
- CABG is recommended in patients ***with symptoms*** of chest pain, shortness of breath, and jaw pain under certain conditions:
  - There is more than 70 percent blockage in one, two, or three of the three arteries *and lifestyle modification and maximum medication-based treatment has already been tried*
  - There is more than 70 percent blockage in one, two, or three arteries *and medication cannot be fully utilized due to other factors or the patient does not want to take medication.*
- Bypass surgery will be harmful, even in patients who have symptoms of chest pain, shortness of breath, and jaw pain, if
  - There is less than 70 percent blockage in the arteries being bypassed.

Overall, *CABG prevents death in around one out of twenty-five patients and prevents a heart attack in around one out of twelve patients.*[21]

What Are the Risks of CABG Surgery?

In the United States, the risk of death after bypass surgery ranges from one in one hundred to one in twenty depending on the total number of surgeries the hospital performs. The more procedures that are performed at a particular hospital, the less risk there is of death due to surgery.

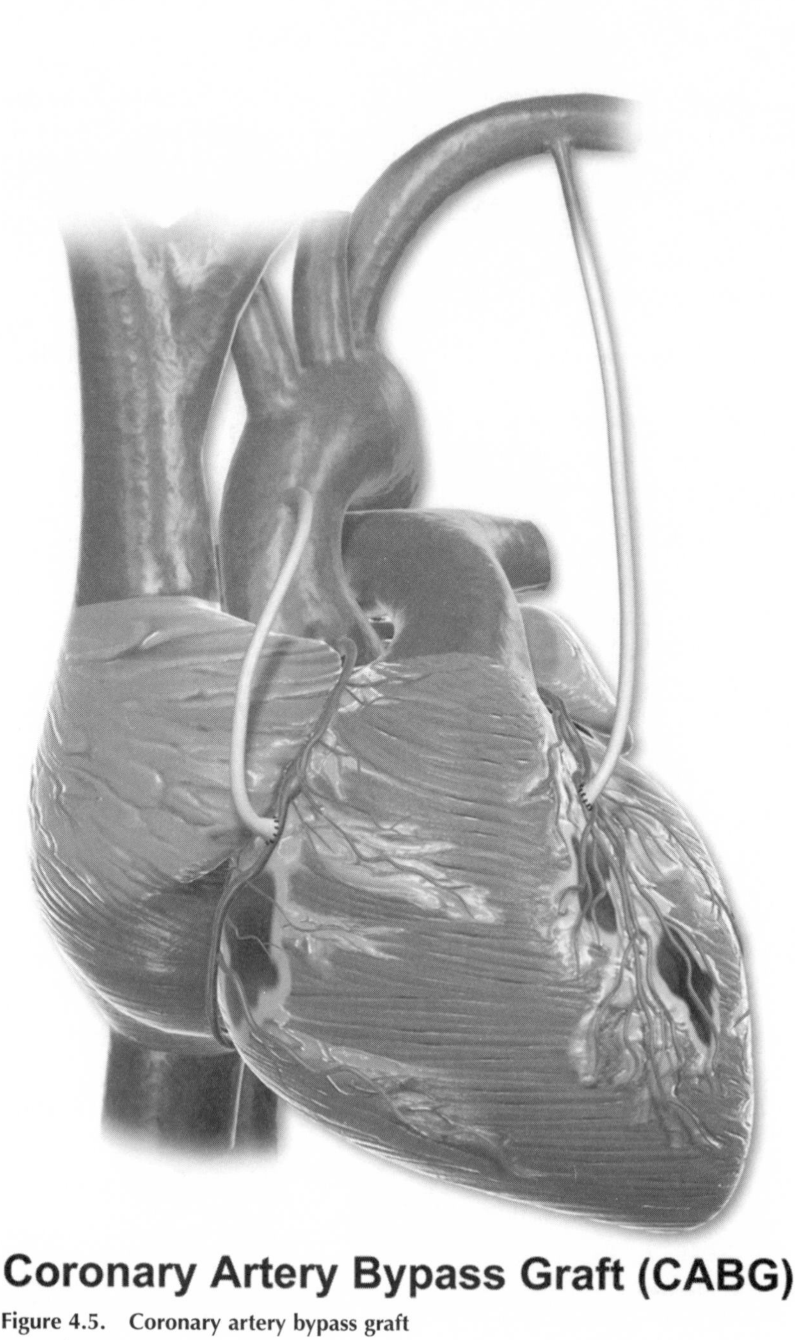

Coronary Artery Bypass Graft (CABG)

Figure 4.5. Coronary artery bypass graft

Bruce Blaus

Not all patients fall into the high-risk category for death due to CABG surgery. However, for those with kidney problems, lung problems, diabetes, poor heart function, and previous cardiac surgery, as well as those who are aged over eighty, the risk of complications will be in the range mentioned above. In these patients it can be especially helpful to understand the benefits and risks of CABG surgery.

Internal bleeding may occur after CABG surgery, and another surgery may be needed in 5 percent of all patients. Strokes can occur in one out of one hundred patients after bypass surgery, and other complications can include:

- Infection of the incision site or internal infection
- The need for reoperation (one in twenty-eight)
- Infection in the blood stream
- Kidney failure (one in forty-three)
- The need for extended life support (one in fourteen)
- Transient heart rhythm problems
- Cognitive decline (one in four).[22]

What Questions Should I Ask my Cardiologist/Cardiac Surgeon before I Consent to CABG?

What Do You Estimate the Blockage to Be in Each Artery?

You need to have *50 percent or greater blockage in the left main artery and 70 percent or more blockage in the other arteries* for it to be considered significant enough to intervene. Once you are informed of what arteries are involved, you can use this information to see if your CABG would be recommended by the American Heart Association guidelines. If not, it may be time to get a second opinion.

Do You Consider Me Symptomatic or Asymptomatic?

This will help you to figure out if you and the surgeon agree on what symptoms you have. If the surgeon says, "Of course you are symptomatic! Don't you have chest pain?" and you don't, it may tell you that

- The doctor does not have all of the correct information about you they need
- The doctor may have an exaggerated sense of how beneficial the surgery will be for you. From here, both of you may be able to come up with an alternative plan.

Some symptoms, such as fatigue or sleepiness, are too vague to be of defini-tive diagnostic use, and it is difficult to determine if these are truly related to blockages in the heart artery or other diseases. Therefore, these types of symptoms may not improve with CABG surgery.

If I Am Asymptomatic, Do You Believe There Is a Survival Benefit to My Having the Surgery?

A doctor can operate to improve your life span or improve your symptoms. If you do not have symptoms and there is no projected improvement to your life span based on your disease profile, then the risk of CABG outweighs the benefit that you may derive from it.

Can Medication Be Tried before We Opt for Surgery?

It is very important to ask this question and will require the cardiologist or surgeon to look at your medication. There is often a rush to surgery. There-fore, once you ask this question, they may pause to consider alternative op-tions. The surgeon will frequently say that they don't know and that it is up to the cardiologist. If they recommend you talk to the cardiologist, do! You will be able to see if there are medications that may hold off surgery. It will also give you more time to consider your options.

How Many Bypass Surgeries Do You and the Hospital Perform Annually?

The more surgeries the surgeon and their team perform, the better off you are. It is important to remember that the rate of death due to CABGs is much higher in hospitals performing less than 150 CABGs per year compared to those performing 450 CABGs per year. The same is true for the average length of hospital stays, as well as the frequency of redo surgery, infection, the need for blood transfusion, and so on.[23]

Can I Wait to Decide on Whether I Want Surgery or Not?

If you walked into the hospital for elective cardiac catheterization, there is no rush to have CABG. Do not let yourself feel like a hostage! Even if the left main artery is blocked 50 percent, it is still possible to wait; this 50 percent blockage did not develop overnight. You have probably had the same level of blockage for the past few weeks or even months! It didn't develop overnight, so it's not progressing overnight.

Cardiologists and surgeons show a considerable urgency to perform CABG surgery when they have patients with left main artery disease, often wanting to get the surgery done on the same day or during the same hospitalization. However, one Polish study found that patients who refused this surgery had similar outcomes at the one-year mark as those who underwent the prescribed procedure.[24] A similar Japanese study followed patients who did not take the doctor's advice for bypass surgery and opted to be treated with medication only. At twelve months, only 5 percent of these patients had succumbed to the disease. This 5 percent is not vastly different from the 4 percent risk of death due to the CABG surgery in high-risk patients.[25] Although it is not advisable to completely refuse the surgery like these patients did, you definitely have enough time to get a second opinion rather than rushing into "emergency" surgery.

Taking a few days to give surgery a second thought and get a second opinion may be worth it in the long run. Furthermore, there is good evidence to show that patients who get elective surgery do much better than those who undergo emergency surgery.

If I Do Not Get the Bypass Surgery, What Is the Chance of My Making It to Next Year? What about the Next Five Years?

Once your doctor has told you how great your blockage is and where it is, you can see where you are in tables 4.1 and 4.2 and decide for yourself what to expect with and without surgery over these time periods.

These are the numbers where CABG makes a difference in survival. For other groups of patients, it does not make a difference compared to medical treatment.

Other Than a Bypass, Will You Be Working on My Valves?

The risk of surgery increases when valves are repaired or replaced. It is very important to know if this additional procedure is going to be performed and, if so, what the repercussions are.

What Is My Risk of Death Thirty Days after Surgery? What about Ninety Days or One Year?

What Are the Other Complications that You Are Worried about in My Case? How Long Will I Stay in the Hospital? Can You or Your Nurse Walk Me Through the STS Calculator So that I Understand My Risks Better?

There is a very good risk calculator from the Society of Thoracic Surgeons that predicts your risk during a CABG procedure based on your age, gender, and medical history. Every patient should expect the surgeon's nurse or nurse practitioner to go over the specific risks of the CABG based on their individual profile.[26] It is critical that you think about the risks so you can take them into account while looking forward to reaping the benefits of the CABG procedure.

Table 4.1. How Many Patients Will Live for Five Years after Heart Condition Is Detected?

Type of heart-artery blockage	Number surviving 5 years with CABG (out of 100)	Number surviving 5 years with medicine but not CABG (out of 100)
3 heart arteries blocked, each > 70%	86	82
Left main artery blocked, > 50%	74	64
Arteries blocked, low heart pumping	80	75

Source: Yusuf et al., "Effect of Coronary Artery Bypass."

Table 4.2. On Average, How Many Months Will Patients with or without CABG Survive?

Type of heart-artery blockage	Average survival after CABG (months)	Average survival with medicine but no CABG (months)
3 heart arteries blocked, each > 70%	104	98
Left main artery blocked, > 50%	100	80
Arteries blocked, low heart pumping	98	88

Source: Yusuf et al., "Effect of Coronary Artery Bypass."

5

Supplements, the Internet, and Heart Monitors: The Customer Has the Controls

SUPPLEMENTS
AKA: NUTRACEUTICALS, HERBAL
PRODUCTS, NATURAL SUPPLEMENTS

One of Those Days

He never would have imagined that he would like cruises, but Jay had enjoyed his vacation with the Royal Caribbean cruise line more than most other vacations he had taken. He had spent most of his time relaxing on the deck, going for nice meals, exercising, and catching up on recent cardiology research. *Sometimes the thought of what you don't have to do gives you the most pleasure*, he thought. Jay was just happy to get away from documenting patient visits, catching up on billing, and attending yet another meeting. Back in medical school nobody had warned him what a big part of his job these tasks would end up accounting for.

But now he was back to the real world! Rested and relaxed, he actually felt keen to take up the medical mantle again. He logged on to the office computer to get the day started. He had apparently done such a good job of switching off that he found he had forgotten his password over the past two weeks and had to use his cheat sheet to retrieve it. The welcome screen listed the patients he would be seeing in the clinic that day. There were some familiar patients and a few new names.

All in a day's work! Jay thought brightly.

Linda, his nurse, walked in holding the first patient chart. She was glad he was back. "Good morning! Did you have a nice vacation, Dr. Johnson?"

"Yes. It was great to get away from it all," Jay said, gesturing to the computer and the pile of papers next to it. "Not having to plan every day of the vacation also felt very good; there was no stress of 'What are we going to do today?' These cruise vacations are fantastic that way."

"Well, you deserved it. Ready for the first patient?" With a grin, she handed him the papers.

Jay nodded and headed to the clinic room.

Common Disease, Uncommon Treatment

The morning's first patient was Abigail, an eighty-three-year-old with high blood pressure and diabetes but normally functioning heart arteries. The pumping of her heart, checked by an echocardiogram, was also normal. About two weeks back she had gone to her family doctor for a routine visit and was found to have atrial fibrillation, an electrical problem in the heart. Abigail was in disbelief over having this problem, since she had been feeling fine. She was continuing to swim three times a week, go on brisk walks with her friends, and take a regular Zumba class. When her family doctor recommended taking a blood thinner, she had become upset; her friend was taking the same blood thinner and had wound up with bruises all over her body. Abigail did not want to be covered in purple spots, and after some back-and-forth, her physician had suggested she talk to a cardiologist.

After reviewing and discussing her history with her, Jay sat down to talk about treatment. The first thing he brought up was blood thinners. "Based on your other risk factors along with the presence of atrial fibrillation, you have about a one in fourteen chance of stroke every year. After much research, we know that we can greatly decrease this risk using one of the blood thinners currently available on the market. Of course, there is a minor increase in the risk of bleeding, but most of these potential bleeds are minor and not life-threatening. Therefore, despite the bleeding risk, the benefit you would gain from blood thinners is tremendous."

"But the atrial fibrillation is gone based on my last test, right? I'm back in normal rhythm?" Abigail asked, protest in her voice.

"Yes, you're in normal rhythm on your EKG," Jay affirmed. "However, we know that once people have had atrial fibrillation they're at increased risk of stroke. That's why we recommend the blood thinner."

"Why do I have to take one? I already bleed easily; if I bump into a table I get a big bruise. I can't imagine what it would be like with the blood thinner as well!"

"I understand your concern; these bruises can be bothersome to a lot of people," Jay empathized. "But can you imagine having a stroke?" he asked, trying his usual lines of argument. "You'd be bedridden and unable to enjoy your life and all the activities you do currently."

"I just don't like taking medicine," she admitted. "I was reading about some natural blood thinners, and I understand that turmeric helps. Can I just use turmeric instead of these medicines? Since it's natural, it's got to be good for me, right?"

Jay scoffed internally. He couldn't resist blurting out, "Arsenic is also natural, but look what happened to everyone who consumed it in the nineteenth century!" He had heard of all the advantages of natural products like turmeric, ginger, and cinnamon and struggled to convince his patients of their medical inefficacy after all the testimonials they had read online.

So, why are doctors opposed to their patients using some of these products? Is there a conspiracy to keep them away from people? Are pharmaceutical companies influencing doctors into prescribing their drugs, luring them with fancy gifts and expensive dinners? Are they all in this together?

Putting It to the Test

It is important to understand how the effectiveness of a certain medical treatment is determined. Over the years, it has been established that a *double-blind placebo-controlled clinical trial* is the best way to assess the effect of a certain treatment.

For example, if we want to assess whether a certain medicine, natural agent, or procedure—here known as *x*—is helpful for a certain disease—here known as *y*—we gather, for example, two hundred patients with disease *y*, giving half of them *x* and the other half either a placebo (usually a sugar pill) or whatever the current established treatment for *y* is. *Both* the patients and the doctors assigned to them are unaware of who has been assigned to get *x* or the placebo or the standard treatment, and so the trial is considered to be *double-blind*. The only party aware of which patients are receiving *x* and which patients are receiving the existing treatment or a placebo is the researcher.

All patients are assessed periodically over the duration of the study, and at the end of a certain time period a final assessment is made to determine which of the two groups faired better. Research studies like these are considered to be the most scientific, valid, and valuable.

So how would science responsibly determine appropriate treatment for a patient like Abigail? One would take two hundred patient-subjects with her similar medical history and put a hundred of them on turmeric and the other hundred on the standard blood thinner for atrial fibrillation. The subjects would then be followed for a certain period—for example, five years. It would then be possible to look over the patients' charts at the close of the study to ascertain how many strokes and how much bleeding occurred in each of the two groups of patient-subjects, determining which treatment was more effective.

But what about all the potential medical benefits of natural supplements and herbs that people like Abigail learn about on the Internet? Is there a double-blind study like this for turmeric?

No.

How about cinnamon?

No.

Perhaps hawthorn?

No.

In light of this, we must ask, are the blood thinners that doctors prescribe held to the highest scientific standards? Are there *double-blind placebo-controlled clinical trials* for these medications?

The use of blood thinners, as it happens, is one of the most researched areas in cardiac care. Numerous double-blind placebo-controlled clinical trials were performed throughout the 1980s and 1990s. Based on several studies like those described above, the use of blood thinners to successfully prevent strokes is well established.[1] The American College of Cardiology gives its highest level of recommendation—known as a *class 1 recommendation*—for starting the blood thinner warfarin (or one of the newer blood thinners) in patients with atrial fibrillation.[2]

If the research is this extensive for well-established treatments and sparse for alternative therapies, how can the average person find out which of these alternative medicines or natural supplements have been assessed and what the results are?

The answer is simple: The nonprofit, nonvendor, government-funded National Center for Complementary and Integrative Health maintains a database on alternative medicines.[3] And "there is little reliable evidence," they say, "to support the use of turmeric for any health condition, because few clinical trials have been conducted."[4]

However, if you search the Internet, you will find many sites that tout the benefits of turmeric and any number of other natural products. But instead of supporting their extensive claims with elaborate, well-designed studies, these vendors of alternative medicine offer perhaps the most prevalent and also most useless kind of proof of their products' effectiveness: testimonials.

While an elaborate story of suffering followed by the discovery of a "miracle" cure is appealing, it is also unscientific and invalid, as details of the patient's unique circumstance and health, critical to any responsible medical analysis, are never provided. Promotional materials often claim that these "treatments" are "doctor-recommended," "the world's most powerful," "patented," or "now presented without a prescription" (even if it had never been prescribed in the first place). These claims are baseless; snake oil by any other name is still snake oil!

But how can you detect these sites and their specious claims? Easy! Every website that touts the benefits of turmeric also has a tab labeled "Cart." Getting your information about turmeric from someone selling it is like asking me if you should buy my book. (The answer is yes, by the way—one copy for each family member and several for your friends as well!)

Whenever you are confronted with claims about the properties of various natural products or supplements, go verify them at the National Center for Complementary and Integrative Health website.

What's in Those Bottles of Natural Products Anyway?

One study by Canadian researchers used DNA sequencing to assess the contents of forty-four herbal products available for sale. They found that one in ten herbal products consisted entirely of fillers and had *no* herbal products at all. One-third of the products had a product *different* from that listed on the label, and about a third also had contaminants not listed on the labels. Overall, *less than half* of the herbal "medicines" for sale actually contained what was listed on the label.[5]

In another study, certain "herbal" antidiabetic products were found to contain undeclared registered or banned oral antidiabetic agents that were to be dispensed and used only under the guidance of physicians. In these cases, patients had been effectively taking diabetes pharmaceuticals without a doctor's prescription or guidance and were thus at risk of being medicated into life-threateningly low blood-glucose levels.[6]

Instances such as these are not uncommon, as the US Food and Drug Administration does not have much regulatory authority over these products. It does not approve or monitor them. The legal requirement expected of the manufacturers of these products is to send a copy of the product label to the FDA, though some do not. Interestingly, a new dietary supplement or formulation can be introduced and marketed overnight even when it contains new, experimental, or unregulated herbal ingredients.[7] These products can be purchased over the counter without a prescription.

But How Can a Natural Product Harm Someone?

With the increased number of patients taking supplements along with their doctor-prescribed drugs[8] comes an increasing possibility of drug interactions. More than half of patients taking supplements are exposing themselves to these dangers. In many cases, doctors are unaware their patients are taking the supplements and cannot advise regarding the possibility of drug interactions.[9]

Some of the problems we have explored that are inherent in today's supplement market—including the sale of products whose actual contents do not match their labels, the potential for drug interaction, and the use of unregulated medications in "herbal" products—can expose patients to harm.[10] It is estimated that twenty-three thousand ER visits each year are related to these supplements.[11] Numerous cases of liver damage result from supplement use, some grave enough to require liver transplants or even resulting in death.[12]

Non-FDA-approved herbal remedies are not covered by insurance plans, and the out-of-pocket cost of these complementary or alternative products is astounding. In 2016 alone the herbal-medicine market was estimated to be worth seventy-one billion dollars. It is estimated to grow to 111 billion dollars by 2023.[13] This does not include the additional cost of visits to alternative providers, which is hardly small change. All of this adds up to significant cost for patients already struggling to pay for health care.

How about the Drugs Doctors Are Prescribing?

The drugs that physicians prescribe undergo rigorous FDA assessment and approval. Any manufacturer who wants to market a drug conducts laboratory tests, animal studies, and clinical trials. They gather information on how effective the drug is, the optimal dosage, the body's response and potential side effects, how long the drug stays in a patient's system, and any potential drug interactions, either with other drugs or with food and drink.

All of this information is then submitted to the FDA. Physicians, statisticians, chemists, pharmacologists, and other scientists at the FDA assess whether or not the information is accurate. Based on these details, they decide if the drug is safe and effective enough for use. If it is considered safe, the drug is then approved for marketing. If it isn't, it is rejected or the manufacturer is asked to collect more information before the drug can be approved.[14]

Overall, these FDA–approved drugs are well researched and rigorously validated. Replacing known, scientifically evaluated, FDA-approved drugs with natural products or supplements can be harmful for several reasons:

- Their unproven efficacy
- Their unregulated content and the potential for adulteration of the product
- The unknown potential for interaction with pharmaceuticals and resulting organ damage
- High out-of-pocket cost.

If you are considering using complementary or alternative medicines, visit the National Center for Complementary and Integrative Health website to check on the current state of scientific evidence on these alternative options first. Please avoid sites that have a button labeled "Cart," as they're likely to be run by unregulated, unmonitored snake oil salesmen. Also, talk to your doctor about any supplements you are considering taking. If you experience any symptoms after starting any alternative supplement along with your prescribed medications, be aware that either of them could be responsible and that it could also be due to an interaction between the two treatments.

It Only Gets Better

Jay took the time to calmly and thoroughly explain why it was medically sound for someone like Abigail to take prescription drug thinners. He knew she was nervous, but it was important and so kept at it, hoping to convince her. In the end, she agreed to read some of the materials he offered her.

"Think about it, and let me know if you want me to prescribe any of the blood thinners I was telling you about." He left her room and looked at his watch. He was already behind by fifteen minutes, and his day was just beginning.

I could use another vacation already, he thought.

As always, Lady Luck averaged it out for him: The next four patients were all doing well, taking their medication, making lifestyle changes, and thriving. There was also a cancellation, so he was left with only one new patient before his lunch break.

Dr. Google and Friends

Jay liked to read up on the details of a patient's medical history before walking into the examination room. It helped him better focus on their concerns during the face-to-face visit. For the next patient, the referring physician's notes had neatly summarized all the information he needed. He would be seeing a twenty-one-year-old man named Chris who had extra beats from the ventricles—*premature ventricular contractions*, or *PVCs*—which had been found incidentally. Chris had no previous medical problems, a normally pumping heart, no blocked arteries, and no valve issues. During the monitoring the family practice doctor had performed, Chris had fifty-eight PVCs in a twenty-four-hour period.

Okay, normal heart with asymptomatic PVCs. No treatment needed. Reassure the kid, and I'm on my way to lunch, Jay thought to himself.

A Very Anxious Patient

However, when he walked in to the examination room, he found Chris and his mother to be in considerable distress. Unfazed, Jay introduced himself and started to get some more details.

"So, Chris, I understand you have some extra beats—PVCs. Tell me, how do you feel when you have these PVCs?"

"That's the problem; I don't feel them. I'm never sure how many I am having, which terrifies me," Chris spoke rapidly, something Jay found common among his patients when they were nervous.

Nodding, Jay hoped that perhaps he had uncovered the reason for Chris's anxiety over this benign condition. "Yes, I understand it can be terrifying. We'll talk about that in a moment. How active are you in general? Do you exercise regularly?"

"I used to, but I've stopped. I don't want to harm myself."

"Hmm," Jay responded thoughtfully. "You think that exercise will harm you?"

"Well, now we know about these PVCs, I'd better be safe. I don't want to worsen them and hurt my heart or be stupid and drop dead."

"You won't drop dead, Chris," Jay tried to reassure him. Chris glanced at his mother, who offered a tentative smile upon hearing that.

"So, you think we can find a way to treat my PVCs and VT? We can do that procedure of zapping the PVCs . . . um . . . ablation, right?" Chris was beginning to sound like a medical student with his use of acronyms and technical jargon.

"I don't think we have to worry about that."

"What do you mean?" Chris asked, seeming puzzled by Jay's devil-may-care attitude.

"PVCs certainly have an impact on your heart function if you have too many of them or have coronary artery disease, weakness of the heart, or a rare genetic disorder. However, you don't have any of those, so the impact is negligible."

"How do you know that I don't have any of that? Isn't that just your assumption?" Chris contested.

"No, I've gone through your medical records. You had an echocardiogram done a week ago, which showed normal heart function. You had a normal stress test, and I've looked at your EKG. All normal."

Jay was doing his best to deescalate the situation, but Chris remained tense and skeptical.

"But those PVCs can turn into runs of VT, and that can lead to sudden death, right?"

Chris's mother looked on in confusion, and Jay looked over at her as he spoke. "PVCs are single extra beats coming from the bottom chamber of the heart. These are abnormal beats. VT, or *ventricular tachycardia*, is beat after beat of these abnormal PVCs, and can cause collapse. Some people die because of this situation."

Chris nodded, glad Jay understood his concerns.

Jay turned his attention to both of them before continuing. "PVCs can lead to VT and sudden death in patients with previous heart attacks, patients with coronary artery disease, or those with cardiomyopathy, or weakness of the heart. However, you do not have any of those conditions, Chris, and so are not at any risk of that. VT can also occur in some rare genetic disorders, but based on your EKG, that doesn't apply to you either. All that reassures me that you are not at risk."

"You don't think these PVCs are going to kill me?"

"I think what we have here is a case of catastrophic thinking. Let me explain what I mean by that: You've convinced yourself that these PVCs are much worse than they actually are—which isn't uncommon when you get medical advice from the Internet. You visit an online chat room, intending to get advice from other people going through the same thing you're going through medically, but in the end all you see are the absolute worst-case scenarios, and you wind up assuming, wrongly, that your own condition is identical to theirs. You end up catastrophizing your situation—getting an inappropriately negative spin on what's actually a benign condition."

At this, Chris's mom found her voice. "I'm so glad you're saying this, Doctor! He's been so upset since reading about all this online."

"But PVCs are abnormal. So how do you explain those? Shouldn't I be tested for genetic disorders?" Chris had read everything he could find online and did not want to leave with any lingering doubts.

"Fifty-eight PVCs per day is not uncommon at all; a lot of people have them. They have no negative impact on your life or health."

"How long can I afford to hold off on exercising? Surely that'll lead to other problems, like gaining weight and being unfit, right?"

"I don't think you have to stop exercising," Jay said. "In fact, the PVCs generally go away when you *are* exercising. During your stress test, you did not have a single PVC. You can start exercising as early as today."

"How about ablation?" Chris asked again. "Do I need to see someone for that?"

"As a physician, I can do two things for any patient: prolong their life in cases where their disease is life-threatening or improve their quality of life if their disease is restraining it. In your case, the PVCs are not life-threatening, so an ablation will not prolong it. Furthermore, you do not have symptoms from these

PVCs, so they're not impacting your quality of life. I cannot make your life any better by chasing them down. Ablation is also an invasive procedure that has the potential to harm you. Based on the guidelines offered by the American College of Cardiology, it would be wrong to perform ablation in your case." Jay was beginning to feel frustrated but made an effort to patiently answer Chris's questions.

"How about a genetic study?"

"There is nothing in your family history that suggests you have a genetic disorder. You do not show any features of one on your EKG either. You don't need a genetic study." Though Jay was measured, he was emphatic. It felt like he was in a candy store with his four-year-old, having to say no multiple times.

"What about an MRI to look for ARVD?"

"ARVD is a rare genetic disorder. Your EKGs are not indicative of ARVD. With no symptoms or EKG abnormality, it's highly unlikely that you have it, so I would strongly advise against an MRI."

Jay was a big advocate of empowering patients with more knowledge about their condition, but he wondered if patients like Chris who read too much on the Internet harm themselves in the long run. Their searches yielded so much information unrelated to their own health condition that they often found it difficult to take in everything Jay was trying to explain to them. Jay would rather write on a blank slate than have to overwrite one filled with nonessential medical jargon.

Paging Dr. Google

Patient education and engagement is a part of medicine cherished by almost everyone. Patients who get involved in their care make more of an effort to stick with their treatment plan and have better health outcomes as a result. Within the limited time allotted to each appointment, physicians try their level best to educate patients. Many physicians' offices offer pamphlets covering a variety of conditions and potential treatment plans. Patients are also encouraged to visit valid websites where authentic, well-researched information can be found, including those of premier institutes such as Mayo Clinic and Cleveland Clinic or professional organizations like the American Heart Association.[15]

However, when patients get their information from unvetted Internet sources, like chat rooms or blog posts, where other patients give information based on their individual experiences, the situation changes. First and foremost, the applicability of the blog or post to the circumstances of each individual reader is questionable. Second, it opens up Pandora's box by going off to irrelevant tangents the reader may not understand or are irrelevant to their medical situation. There is a distinct possibility that reader's anxiety will be increased over something they may not even need to worry about. Ratcheting up patient concern over irrelevant matters makes face-to-face time with the physician less efficient and increases the likelihood that the patient will be subjected to increased testing to put to rest unnecessary concern about rare diseases or conditions evoked by spurious, unfounded, or inapplicable information found online.[16]

There are also many sites that promote certain procedures or devices used in particular conditions. It is necessary to be aware of the commercial bias present in those cases. A young-looking sixty-five-year-old may be shown to have a perfect life after receiving a particular device or procedure. Unfortunately, the same treatment may not provide similar benefits to an eighty-five-year-old with dementia, a hip replacement, poorly controlled diabetes, and lung disease. The applicability of the various treatment plans to an individual patient can best be assessed by a meticulous physician performing due diligence and taking into consideration the patient's overall clinical condition.

Many apps and websites offer diagnoses based on the analysis of patient symptoms. Although these may prove helpful in some cases, they generally do a poorer job than would a physician's evaluation. In a study comparing the two, physicians outperformed the automated, algorithm-based websites by a wide margin.[17] Though at some point in the future technologies like these may play an important supporting role in patient care, they are not ready to replace doctors yet.

Lunch Time and Beyond

Over lunch, Jay had a good conversation with his fellow cardiologists about their upcoming travel plans. Three of the five of them had traveled far and wide, while the other two had vacation homes where they spent most of their off time. When the conversation turned to which websites offered the best online fares, Jay mentioned the issue of patients searching the Internet for medical advice.

It seemed that the group was of two minds about it: Some appreciated their patients' involvement in their care. That said, all of them were wary of patients like Chris who read every mention of their condition in online chat rooms and blog posts. None of Jay's colleagues could offer a solution for managing the flow of the crucial elements of conversation when patients came to them with a large amount of irrelevant or misleading information.

After his break, Jay returned to the clinic, refreshed. The first two patients of the afternoon were well known to him and just in for follow-ups. He was encouraged by the lifestyle changes they had made. One of them had been tobacco-free for five months, while his eighty-year-old patient had recovered from heart valve surgery and was now walking two or three miles a day. He was upbeat when his nurse brought him the details for the next patient.

"Not much here," she said, handing him a single piece of paper.

"A new patient with no records?" Jay was puzzled.

"No past history, no recorded meds, no history of allergies, nada!" Linda proclaimed. "They're self-referred."

"Huh!" Jay was always curious about these self-referred patients. They made an appointment to see a cardiologist directly, bypassing family physicians and primary care physicians, and often had intriguing stories.

The Quantified Self: Another Day, Another Technophile

Jay introduced himself to the patient, a young forty-five-year-old man. He appeared to be fit and well-dressed and had his company ID still dangling from his belt. *Jared Murphy, Director of Information Systems*, the badge read.

"So, I don't have any information about you or your past medical history," said Jay. "Tell me, what brings you to a cardiologist's office at this young age?"

"Well," said the man, "it seems that I have a cardiac problem, but I'm not sure what it is."

Jay smiled. "That's job security for me, right?" He hoped his light-hearted quip wouldn't be misunderstood.

Jared smiled back in good humor and continued. "I am concerned about my heart rate and wondering what's wrong."

Jay's heart sank as he sensed where this was going.

Jared pointed to his wristwatch. "I have a new smartwatch I got for my birthday, and I've been using it to track my heart rate during my weekend bicycle rides for the past two months. I've noticed I'm going way above my target heart rate within moments of exercising, and I have to go really slow to remain in the range. But that impacts my training; I'm gearing up for a hundred-mile ride this summer."

"How do you feel while training? Are you getting out of breath or experiencing any chest pain or dizziness?"

"No, no problems at all; I don't feel any of that. I did this same bicycle ride last year, and I was fine, and I feel like I'm in better shape than I was last year. I've been riding fifty to sixty miles every weekend and feeling good. I don't know why my heart rate jumps up so quickly to 180 bpm when my target heart rate is 175. Trying to remain below the target heart rate means having to slow waaaay down. What kind of testing should we do?"

Delaying a response, Jay continued his clinical line of questioning. "Are you losing weight? Gaining weight?"

"Nope. Steady as always," Jared responded.

"How's your hydration level? Are you keeping well-hydrated during your training rides?"

"Yes. I carry a gallon of water with me and keep myself hydrated."

"Okay. Do you know how your heart rate recovery is?"

"It's in the normal zone. My heart rate recovers to normal within six minutes of ending my ride."

"Yes, that is normal," Jay confirmed. "I understand from the papers you filled out that you don't have any other medical conditions and you haven't had any surgeries. Is that right?"

"Yes—I've always been healthy and fit. I occasionally suffer from seasonal allergies, but nothing beyond that."

"If you aren't having any symptoms and your heart rate is recovering well, I don't think we need to worry about your heart rate being above the target rate set by the formula," Jay reassured him. "You should continue to train by listening to your body. If you feel fine, continue to push yourself."

"You don't think I should do a stress test to see if I have blockages?"

"If you're not having any symptoms while exercising to this level, I'm not sure a stress test would be of any value. This is particularly true for you, since you have no family history of blockages in the heart arteries, no risk factors like high blood pressure or diabetes, and you have been a nonsmoker all your life." Jay was grateful that the paperwork had been so minimal, as he'd been able to remember everything.

"But what's the explanation behind there being such a quick jump to the target heart rate? A stress test could clarify things, correct?"

"Just like height and weight, one's target heart rate is a range, not an exact number," Jay said. "There's considerable variation in how different people's heart rates react to exercise. The target heart rate formula holds true for a *group* of individuals. Yes, in a large group of forty-five-year-olds, the average maximum heart rate may be 175 beats per minute. However, within that group there's substantial variation from one person's target heart rate to another. Heart rate also changes depending on many factors, such as your sleep, the weather, or your training level. Therefore, even in the same person, there can be perfectly normal variation from one day to another."

Jared still looked doubtful. "Is there any harm in doing a stress test to check it out?"

"Yes, actually, there is," Jay said. "Your chance of having a heart blockage as a forty-five-year-old with no risk factors is around seven in a thousand. With your level of exercise and lack of symptoms added in, the chances of finding a blockage in the heart artery are likely to be closer to seven in ten thousand. At that level, doing a stress test is not only unhelpful but probably harmful. The American College of Cardiology does not recommend stress testing in situations like this."

After another fifteen minutes of conversation and fielding questions, Jay was able to convince Jared of his well-being. He wondered if it would have helped telling Jared the real story behind target heart rates.

The Science Behind the Maximum Heart Rate

By the late 1960s, physicians had recognized the value of exercise and fitness and had been recommending a moderate amount of exercise to their patients. However, they did not have any numbers that they could ask the patients to adhere to.

The federal public-health service had a heart-disease program, whose staff included Drs. Samuel Fox and William Haskell, among others. In 1970, these doctors were asked to give recommendations regarding how strenuously a *patient with heart disease* could safely exercise. According to Dr. Haskell's account, he selected information from about ten published studies of cardiac patients who were below the age of fifty-five and likely to be smokers. He assessed their maximum heart rate in these studies. As they were flying to their meeting, making last-minute preparations, Dr. Haskell pulled out his data and shared it with Dr. Fox. They observed the maximum heart rate in different age groups and drew a line through the graph of averages.

"Gee," Dr. Haskell observed, "if you extrapolate that out, it looks like at age twenty the heart rate maximum is two hundred, at age forty it's 180, and at age sixty it's 160."

And so Dr. Fox suggested a very rough formula to determine maximum heart rate:

$$\text{maximum heart rate} = 220 - \text{age}$$

Both doctors, of course, recognized that there was large variation among individuals from these averages. For a given age, if the formula estimated that the target heart rate was 180 beats per minute, there were also people with a maximum recorded heart rate of 210 beats per minute and some with 150 beats per minute. However, they wanted to provide a simple guideline *for cardiac patients* and so settled on the single formula.[18]

Maximum Heart Rate Takes On a Life of Its Own

Despite these limitations, Drs. Fox and Haskell's formula quickly entered medical literature, eventually trickling down to the general population. Doctors now had an easy number to give all their patients, and the formula that had been hastily derived based on patients with heart diseases now took on the weight of scientific certitude. Doctors, exercise gurus, gymnasiums, and others promoted the formula so often that it became entrenched. Graphs were posted on the walls of health clubs and cardiology treadmill rooms, reprinted in textbooks, and marketed to cardiac patients and healthy people alike.*[20]

As so frequently happens, certain entrepreneurial minds saw an opportunity, and the heart-rate-monitoring industry took off. Wearable devices measuring heart rates were invented, and running magazines, running clubs, and manufacturers promoted them. Even casual weekend runners now felt obligated to purchase one of the seemingly ubiquitous heart rate monitors.[21]

The market for these devices grew by leaps and bounds. According to one report, more than seventeen million wearable devices, including smart watches and fitness bands, were purchased in 2014 alone. Projections estimated that in 2017 forty-five million of these gadgets would be sold.[22]

Are Fitness Trackers Useful and Reliable?

There is no doubt that heart rate monitors may help motivate people who are numbers-driven. Additionally, they may provide pertinent data for patients with certain rare heart conditions. However, for the average person, the value of regularly monitoring heart rate is limited.[23] Think of target heart rate as you would think about height: Just as there is no single normal height but a range of normal heights, there is no single maximum heart rate for healthy individuals of a certain age. "Normal" is only a range—and a very wide range at that!

There are many heart rate monitors currently available on the market. Most of them perform better at rest than during moderate activity, which raises the question of reliability. Given this, scientists who study these gadgets believe that there is inadequate research about the usefulness of activity-tracker data. So, doctors cannot advise patients about certain health issues based on these gadgets alone.[24]

However, the obsession with tracking using heart rate monitors has gone too far. Some physicians have expressed concerns that among the general population the unnecessary and persistent tracking of heart rates is spreading.[25] Increasing numbers of users compare their personal data to the standard and, like Jared, conclude that anything below or above that standard indicates a medical

---

* Years later when looking back, Dr. Haskell, now a professor at Stanford University, said, "I've kind of laughed about it over the years. The formula was never supposed to be an absolute guide to rule people's training. It's so typical of Americans to take an idea and extend it beyond what it was originally intended for."[19]

problem, making them anxious. If there is reliable data and a reasonable level of concern under the right circumstances, deviation from the normal range may need to be assessed. However, most of the time considerable amounts of effort and resources are spent on unnecessary tests that follow abnormal findings on these gadgets. These tests are of little actual value to the patient's health.[26]

The Bottom Line

Dr. Gerald Fletcher, professor of medicine at Mayo Clinic, gave the final word on the issue: "The majority of people simply don't need to monitor their heart rate."[27]

But if monitoring is unnecessary, what is the best strategy for exercise?

According to Edward F. Coyle, PhD, professor of kinesiology and health education at the University of Texas at Austin and director of the university's Human Performance Laboratory, "If you're exercising for health, the most important thing to do is get off the couch." For most people, he adds, the key is simply to "enjoy their exercise, so they keep doing it."[28]

6

Pacemakers: A Surefire Spark?

It isn't that they cannot find the solution. It is that they cannot see the problem.

—Attributed to G. K. Chesterton

PACEMAKERS

That Time of the Year

Patricia had insisted that everyone come home for Thanksgiving this year. For the past few years, her two children had taken turns hosting the family, but she wanted to prepare the feast at home, the way she liked it, and was too tired to endure crowded airports. The children had agreed, but they'd insisted she not go overboard with preparation.

Carla and her family arrived on Wednesday, while Peter and his wife landed on a red-eye Thursday morning. Patricia was relieved they had all made it on time and thrilled to have her children back under one roof. Once Peter arrived, Carla made coffee, and they all sat around the kitchen table, sipping, chatting about their year.

"How about yours, Mom? You've been pretty quiet," Carla said, nudging Patricia.

"Oh, you know. It's the same old, same old here," Patricia said dismissively.

"How is your friend Boris? Are you two still in the bowling league?" Peter asked.

"Oh, no, dear! I haven't gone bowling for a while, and I haven't seen Boris recently."

"Oh . . . Are you still volunteering at the library? How many Volunteer of the Year awards are you up to now?"

"I go there once in a while, but not as much as I used to," Patricia replied quietly, seeming subdued.

Peter and Carla exchanged a worried glance. She was acting now like she had that first year after their dad's death; but even then she had bounced back well. For the past seven years, she had been thriving socially. But before they could press her further, she rose, and they all got busy preparing Thanksgiving dinner. Peter ran to the grocery store, and Carla stayed back to help Patricia cook.

As Carla opened the refrigerator, she noticed the magnet her father had loved—*I hope I don't outlive my mind.* Carla briefly paused, recalling how his wish had been granted by the fatal heart attack that had taken him in his sleep.

Carla was surprised to find the refrigerator well stocked with preprepared dinner packages; Patricia had always been proud of her role as home cook when they were growing up. "Somebody's taken a liking to frozen dinners! I didn't know you were into Lean Cuisine®, Mom."

"It's much easier for just one person. Less cleaning."

They continued their preparations, but after just fifteen minutes Patricia excused herself to go lie down for a bit. Carla scurried around getting dinner ready, but as she moved through the kitchen, rifling through drawers and hunting through the pantry shelves, she realized that many essentials were missing. She had to keep texting Peter to pick up yet another thing from the store.

When Peter returned an hour later, Carla seemed stressed.

"Where's Mom?" he asked. "She left you in the kitchen by yourself?"

"She went to take a nap soon after you left. Come help me in here; I can't seem to find the baking soda."

"Finally, she trusts us in the kitchen by ourselves!" Peter said as they rummaged through the cupboards, looking for the ingredients. "Talk about a turnaround, eh?"

"I don't know. I've never known her to take a nap—and at eleven in the morning? I'm beginning to worry."

"Well, maybe she's just feeling under the weather."

"I don't know," she said again. "I keep thinking of last year. She was doing all the cooking—taking over my kitchen, chopping, preparing, cleaning, doing everything. Something's off."

"Okay, we can talk about it later. Tell me what needs to be done here."

They busied themselves in the kitchen, though Peter had to run out a couple more times to pick up yet more missing ingredients.

After a couple of hours, Patricia joined Carla. The dinner they managed to prepare wasn't going to be as elaborate a feast as Patricia had made in years past. It turned out fine, though Patricia seemed quiet throughout the meal. She didn't seem to notice that their traditional brussels sprout casserole was missing. The change from last year was very pronounced. It continued to bother Carla.

Later, they all settled in the living room. Carla sat on the couch beside Patricia and brought up her concerns about the packaged dinners, the nap, the missing essentials in the kitchen . . . Patricia brushed them off with excuses, saying she felt tired all the time, but dismissing the fatigue as a part of getting older. After Patricia went to bed, Carla again voiced her worries to Peter.

"I agree with you, Carla—something's off. She was quiet all through dinner and hardly said anything to the kids. She's not her usual self."

"Is it usual for people her age to be tired all the time?" Carla hoped Peter's previous job as an EMT could help them pinpoint what was wrong.

"Is that what she said? She's tired all the time?"

"Yeah, but as a side note, you know? Dismissing it as age-related. She was trying to change the subject."

Peter thought that was concerning, and they decided to discuss it again with Patricia the next day.

*   *   *

The next morning, Patricia woke up later than usual. Over coffee, Peter and Carla talked to her about her fatigue. Her responses did not reassure them.

"I've stopped exercising for a while," Patricia confessed. "I just don't feel like it anymore." She said she had not discussed these changes with anyone, including her doctors.

Peter and Carla felt guilty about not having connected with her more throughout the year; they wish they had known about this sooner. But now they were here and wanted to address the issue as soon as possible, before they left, going back to their own lives. The office of Dr. Saleh, the family doctor, was closed that day, so instead they brought Patricia to urgent care.

It was a little busy, but the nurse soon checked them into a room. She started asking a laundry list of questions while taking Patricia's temperature, blood pressure, and pulse rate. She rechecked the pulse rate on the other arm, as if she didn't believe the first reading.

"Your pulse rate is low. Have you always had a low pulse?" she asked.

"Yes; they don't think it's a big deal," Patricia replied.

The nurse nodded slowly and filled out the rest of the form before leaving the room. "The doctor will be right in."

But five minutes later she was back, with an EKG machine. "Your pulse rate is forty-eight beats a minute, which is low. The doctor has asked for an EKG," she explained. She put some stickers on Patricia's chest, had her lie back, and after a few minutes got an EKG printout. She left the room once more, presumably to hand it to the doctor.

Within a minute, the doctor walked in, EKG in hand.

"So, you're here because of fatigue, right?" he asked, reading from the nurse's papers.

"She's been unusually tired," Carla interjected.

"For how long?"

"A few months—right, Mom?" Carla continued to answer for Patricia, who just nodded.

"I think we may have an answer," the doctor said. "We'll perform more tests and get some blood work done, but your heart rate is very low. Forty-eight beats a minute can make anyone tired. Are you on any medication?" he asked, leafing through the other paperwork the nurse had filled out. Before they could answer, he continued, "Only calcium for bones—nothing else?" He was clearly in a rush.

"Yes," Patricia said.

"I think we need to transfer you to the hospital. You need a pacemaker," he concluded.

"Why a pacemaker? And—"

Before Carla could finish, the doctor's cell phone rang, and he walked out to take the call. Within a few minutes, a flurry of activity arose around Patricia. Carla asked to talk to the doctor again, but her request fell on deaf ears. Everyone was busy arranging Patricia's urgent transfer to the hospital.

The family could not ask any questions or think through the process. They hoped that they would get a chance to do so at the hospital.

A Speedy Hospital Admission

At the hospital, Patricia was sent to the holding area, where she was prepared for the pacemaker procedure. Peter and Carla stood back, allowing the nurses and other staff to start working on their mom, placing an IV line, drawing blood for some tests, and, of course, asking all the questions needed to fill out the paperwork. Soon Patricia was given some forms to sign.

A nurse explained what each form was for.

"Here—this next form is giving permission for Dr. Rose to put in the pacemaker. Go ahead and sign this." Her monologue sounded well practiced.

"I think we'd like to talk to the cardiologist before signing it," Carla broke in. "We have no idea why this is needed; Mom was just shifted from urgent care to out here and told she needs a pacemaker. We have no idea what's wrong!"

"Okay then," said the nurse. "We will wait for Dr. Rose." She seemed irritated about being stopped midflow. Soon she brought out two wires and a gadget the size of two quarters stacked together. "Two wires like these will go inside your heart," she said, addressing Patricia, "and then get attached to this device, which is the battery. The battery will go underneath the skin here," she pointed to Patricia's left shoulder. All three nodded, understanding what was to come. But they still didn't understand *why* Patricia needed this pacemaker.

We Have the Answer

After about forty-five minutes, Dr. Rose arrived, holding Patricia's EKG, and introduced himself. He seemed an experienced cardiologist, though maybe he'd neglected to heed the oft-repeated advice about exercise.

"You've been feeling very tired for the past few months, yes, and are taking frequent naps?" he began. "You have had some dizziness while standing up and are not on any heart medicine," he summarized from the notes, appearing to know all the relevant details.

The group nodded, and he continued. "Your EKG shows you have slow heartbeats. The electrical system of your heart is aging; it has nothing to do with blockages in the heart arteries or anything like that. There's no need for stents, angioplasty, or bypass surgery, but the electrical wires of your heart have been frayed, so to speak, so you have a slow heart rate."

He paused briefly to make sure they understood, then continued. "At forty-eight beats a minute, you're not getting enough blood to your brain or your body. As a result, you're feeling tired. A pacemaker will give you a high enough heart rate to get sufficient blood flow to your body. It should take away the fatigue, and you may not need to take as many naps."

He had provided the best explanation they'd gotten so far, and they were grateful for it. Carla and Peter were relieved their mom would soon start feeling better and hopefully return to her old self.

Pushing a form across the table for Patricia to sign, Dr. Rose said, "This is just the consent form. Once you sign it, we can start the procedure. You'll feel 100 percent better after you have this pacemaker."

Patricia looked over to her children, who nodded their approval. She signed the paper, and the final preparations were underway. Before long, she was wheeled out of the room, ready for her pacemaker procedure, and Carla and Peter were asked to move to the family waiting area.

"I'm so glad we brought her to urgent care," Carla breathed, as the two of them walked out.

"Yeah! I wonder how long she would have carried on struggling if we hadn't insisted on bringing her." Peter knew his mother well.

"She'll be back to Energizer Bunny mode after this pacemaker," Carla said, hopefully. "Interesting technology, isn't it? Who knew such a small gadget could have such a great impact?" She wondered about the marvels of modern medicine that had made these magical gadgets such a routine part of life.

A Spark for the Heart

The heart has fascinated mankind throughout history; even the Greek philosopher Aristotle wrote extensively about its relevance and structures. However, the electrical system of the heart wasn't discovered for more than two millennia after his death. In 1887, British physician Augustus Waller was the first to record electrical activity in the human heart, using a capillary electrometer, a precursor to the modern EKG.

But Augustus was pessimistic about its use. "I do not imagine that electrocardiography is likely to find very extensive use in the hospital," he said. "It can at most be of rare and occasional use to afford a record of some rare anomaly." Over the next fifty years, he was proven wrong, as electrocardiography evolved and came into routine use.[1]

By the 1930s, American physician Albert Hyman had observed that a stopped heart could be made to beat by inserting a needle into it. He connected this needle to a spring wound hand-cranked motor. Electrical impulses from the motor could now be transmitted to the heart in a rhythmic manner by the needle. He called his device an *artificial pacemaker*. Unfortunately, the medical community dismissed Hyman's work, and major journals refused to publish his findings.

In the 1950s, the spring-wound hand-cranked motor was replaced with the alternating current from an electrical socket. This advancement updated the technology but left the patient's mobility limited to only a short distance from electrical sockets. This, among many other limitations, restricted the use of this device, and once again the innovation was ignored by the medical community. An artificial pacemaker that could be implanted inside the patient, complete with its own electric supply, would be crucial to making this technology acceptable.[2] It would take a fortunate blunder to make this marvel of modern medicine a reality!

The Mistake that Saved a Million Lives

Wilson Greatbatch was born in 1919 to English immigrants, and named in honor of then-president Woodrow Wilson. As a teenager, growing up in Buffalo, New York, Wilson was fascinated by radio technology, and so after high school, he joined the armed forces, and went on to become an aviation chief radioman. Once discharged from the military, he married and began work as a telephone repairman. It wasn't long before he decided to pursue his interest further, earning a degree in electrical engineering at Cornell University in 1950. New diploma in hand, he took a job as a manager in the electronics division at the Taber Instrument Corporation.[3]

At the time of his accidental breakthrough that would come to redefine modern medical treatment, Wilson was working on a device that recorded heart rhythm. He described his serendipitous discovery in the following way: "The oscillator required a ten thousand–ohm resistor at the transistor base. I reached into my resistor box for one, but I misread the color coding and got a one-megohm resistor by mistake."[4]

When he plugged in this resistor, the circuit *gave rather than recorded* an electrical impulse. The gadget emitted an electrical pulse rhythmically for 1.8 milliseconds, followed by a one second break. He stared at the gadget in disbelief; it was replicating the heart rhythm! Years before, while discussing the natural electrical circuitry of the heart, he had learnt that rhythmic electrical stimulation followed by a break could replace a malfunctioning heart rhythm. And now he was watching precisely that stimulation being given off by his two-cubic-inch gadget. He immediately realized its potential. His serendipitous finding would be able to rhythmically stimulate the human heart using these sequences of electrical pulse. The gadget could mimic the heart's electrical system.

He labored to finish his prototype and brought it to the animal lab at the Veterans' Hospital in Buffalo, where he knew the surgeons through his work. In order to assess the gadget, the chief of surgery, Dr. Chardack, exposed the heart of a dog. He and another surgeon touched the two wires of the gadget to the heart, which immediately started beating in synchrony with the device. They looked at each other in disbelief. "Well, I'll be damned!" said Dr. Chardack, speaking for everyone in the room.[5]

Wilson was over the moon. He later said, "I seriously doubt if anything I ever do will give me the elation I felt that day, when a two-cubic-inch electronic device of my own design controlled a living heart."[6]

His company, Taber Instrument Corporation, did not want to invest their resources in this new gadget, but Wilson understood its potential. He decided to take a chance and dedicate his full attention to its development. Relying on his vegetable garden and savings of two thousand dollars to feed his family, he gave up his job. Over the next two years, he perfected the prototype in a barn behind his home. Teaming up with Dr. Chardack, he demonstrated the device's efficacy in dogs over the months that followed, and soon the artificial pacemaker was patented.[7]

In June 1960, Chardack and his surgical team implanted the first pacemaker in a seventy-seven-year-old man suffering complete electrical failure of the heart. By the end of 1960, the pacemaker had been implanted in ten patients, including two children. In 1961, Dr. Chardack reported their experience with this device among a series of fifteen patients.[8] The device was licensed to Medtronic that same year. On the strength of the use of these pacemakers, Medtronic quickly became a world leader in medical electronics.[9]

Technology Evolves

Pacemakers have continued to evolve over the last half century. The initial obscure and clunky technology is gone, and they can now be implanted via a small incision in the skin, running on small batteries lasting up to twelve years.

Every age group has benefitted from pacemakers. In the United States, millions of people currently live normal lives thanks to this marvelous technology. Hundreds of thousands of elderly patients have been able to live longer and better-quality lives due to their pacemakers, thousands of infants have been saved from certain death, and newborns have received pacemakers as early as fifteen minutes after birth to save their lives.[10] Many patients have fulfilled their lifelong dreams of running marathons and climbing mountains thanks to pacemakers.[11]

One landmark study of Dutch patients noted that when the right patients get a pacemaker for the right reason, their heart's electrical system is taken over by the pacemaker. From that point on, their health outcome is similar to those who have not had any malfunction of the cardiac electrical system at all.[12]

Considering the procedure's phenomenal worldwide success, it would be natural to believe that Patricia would soon join the ranks of millions whose lives were improved by pacemakers.

Patricia Has the Pacemaker

After about an hour, Dr. Rose came out to the waiting room, where he found Carla and Peter, surprising them with the speed of the procedure. "It all went well; your mom has the pacemaker fitted," he began, smiling but brisk. "She'll stay overnight, but tomorrow morning, she can go home. Alright?" He left before they could ask any questions.

As expected, Patricia was discharged the next day with instructions on how to care for the wound. She was told to not to raise her left arm or lift any weight for a month. This would mean seriously curtailing her day-to-day activity, so Peter decided to stay back to help out his mother.

Hopes of Turning a Corner

In the days after the surgery, Peter noticed that his mom continued to fatigue easily. He checked her pulse routinely, almost obsessively. It was always around sixty beats per minute when she was sitting down, but she continued to take naps every midmorning. At the one-week post-op checkup at the doctor's office, the nurse assured them the wound was healing well.

"Why is she tired all the time?" Peter asked as the nurse checked the pacemaker function.

"It's probably from the anesthesia," she told him, not taking her eyes from the laptop-like device she was fiddling with. "As people age, they don't bounce back from surgeries as quickly as they used to. Give it a bit of time." After a few minutes of punching buttons and checking the screen, she concluded, "The pacemaker is working well. The wires are remaining in place, and all the numbers are perfect." Before she left the office, she repeated all the dos and don'ts Patricia needed to follow over the next three weeks.

* * *

For the next week or so, there wasn't much of a change in Patricia's energy levels. Peter would go for regular evening walks with her, but he noticed that within twenty minutes she would be too tired to go further. This was surprising, as she'd once been very active. She'd been a runner all her life, registering for local 10ks up until just the year prior. So for her not to be able walk at a gentle pace for even half an hour? Peter decided something was terribly wrong.

When he told Carla about it over the phone, she too was taken aback. "Can you get her back in to see Dr. Rose? Ask him when we can expect her to bounce back."

"Yeah, I called his office yesterday. She has an appointment to see him next week."

"Okay, I'll talk to him about it." Carla was already planning to spend two weeks out there to relieve Peter, and she would accompany her mom to the appointment.

When Carla arrived, she saw what her brother was talking about with the fatigue, but she also noticed other changes. Patricia often failed to recall the events of the day before and would occasionally struggle to find words. Carla couldn't wait to get some answers about this from Dr. Rose.

A Quick Visit

On the day of the appointment, Carla made sure she wrote down all her questions for Dr. Rose ahead of time. She didn't want to waste this clinic visit.

"How have you been? Is your fatigue better? Walking more, taking fewer naps?" the doctor asked.

"I am alright," Patricia responded.

Carla shook her head, "No, Mom. You are still tired." She turned to Dr. Rose, "Mom continues to take naps."

"Well," Dr. Rose continued, poring over her chart, "the pacemaker is working well. All the numbers are good, the wires are remaining in position, and she's getting all the heartbeats her body needs." He looked through the notes as he spoke.

"But how about her fatigue? We thought the pacemaker would make it better. That's why she was brought here from urgent care; they said it was because of the slow heartbeats. But now the heartbeats are normal, right?" Carla could not hide her frustration.

"I'm not sure why she's tired; we may need to look elsewhere for the cause. Talk to her primary care physician about it," said Dr. Rose. "Her pacemaker is working well; her heart is fine," he emphasized. "There may be other things causing the fatigue."

Carla realized that the list of questions that she had written down was worthless; he would not be answering any of them. She would have to talk to Dr. Saleh, her mother's primary care physician.

A Healthy Long-Term Relationship

Over the past twenty years, they had never had difficulty getting in to see Dr. Saleh. Sure enough, within three days Patricia was able to see her. Carla had her list of questions ready.

"How have you been?" asked Dr. Saleh warmly.

Carla realized that Dr. Salah always asked open-ended questions and gave ample time for response. This was a welcome change.

"I got this thing here . . . pacemaker?" Patricia responded, looking at Carla for confirmation.

Dr. Saleh was surprised. "Oh, what happened? Nobody told me about it."

Carla looked confused for a moment. "They said they would send you the reports. They didn't?" She went on to relay the complete story of Patricia's fatigue over Thanksgiving, the visit to urgent care, Patricia's slow heart rate, and then the pacemaker.

"How slow was the heart rate? Do you recall?" Dr. Saleh inquired.

"Uh . . . forty-eight, I think." Carla was surprised she remembered the number.

Dr. Saleh started going back and forth through the chart she held. Other than the ruffling of papers, there was silence. After a couple of minutes, she said, "She has always had a low heart rate, but it has never been an issue. It is slow because your mother has performed vigorous aerobic activities throughout her life. Didn't she compete in high school?"

"Yes, and she continued with long-distance running up until last year," Carla responded. She was confused as to what Dr. Saleh was implying.

"All her records from the past indicate a low pulse rate. We even tested her with a twenty-four-hour monitor three years ago. Her heart rate dropped to forty beats a minute at night, but she has never been troubled by it," the doctor explained. "It has never been a threat to her health or life. We have talked about it, haven't we, Patricia?"

"So why is she tired? Isn't it because of her low heart rate?"

"I don't think so. People who have been runners or bicyclists have a low heart rate and aren't bothered by it. Has the pacemaker helped? Have her energy levels improved?"

"No, it doesn't seem to have made much of a difference." Carla admitted. "She's still tired, and they tell us that the pacemaker is working well. That's what I wanted to talk to you about."

"Unfortunately, finding the cause of symptoms is not always straightforward. Fatigue can be caused by many different health issues, including low blood count, sleep deprivation, and depression, as well as low heart rate. We have to explore each possible cause of fatigue and see which one applies in her case," Dr. Saleh explained.

"Why did they not do this before putting in the pacemaker?" Carla couldn't hide her frustration.

"Well," Dr. Saleh sighed.

"I know you weren't involved in the decision making, but it's surprising that they rushed in with a pacemaker," Carla continued to vent.

Dr. Saleh nodded. Then, as if apologizing for the system, she added, "Sometimes once a certain diagnosis has taken hold, the thinking process stops. It is a cognitive error called *premature closure* where doctors do not consider reasonable alternatives once they have made a diagnosis. It is unfortunately a common cause of misdiagnosis in medicine.[13] Once they decided that the heart rate was linked to her fatigue, they did not assess other symptoms that she had, nor did they look at other possible causes of her fatigue. I am sorry she had to go through this."

Carla was touched by how open Dr. Saleh was talking about errors that can happen in health care. Dr. Saleh took the time to discuss with her the possible causes for Patricia's low energy, tests to run, and specialists to see. This seemed like a much more sensible and smart approach than the rush with the pacemaker, Carla noted. She couldn't help thinking of a quip she'd heard somewhere before: *What's the difference between a general practitioner and a specialist? One treats what you have, the other thinks you have what he treats!*

Why was it Patricia got a pacemaker in such a rush? The technology has definitely saved a lot of lives and improved the quality of life for millions, so was this a rare case of poor judgment?

Spreading like Wildfire

In the initial years after the first pacemaker implants, only a handful of physicians were able to perform the procedure. This new technology saved many lives throughout the 1960s but was fraught with problems. Sometimes the wires failed, occasionally the battery drained suddenly, and frequently other technical issues arose. Few physicians felt comfortable putting in pacemakers because of these problems, so the industry collaborated with them to solve these critical issues.[14]

Over the next few years, the technology for the wires improved, becoming more reliable, and now they could be placed via the veins into the heart. The battery technology also advanced, becoming more reliable and longer-lasting. The size of the pacemakers also reduced, and nonsurgical cardiologists could soon fit them.[15]

These advances led to greater acceptance of the procedure. Approval of payment for the pacemaker procedure by Medicare provided an additional boost, and it was soon recommended for a wider variety of diseases. The rate of placement of pacemakers increased by 45 percent annually over the 1960s, and from a few dozen pacemakers being implanted early in the decade, the total grew to ten thousand by 1967. By the early 1980s, over one hundred thousand new pacemakers were placed in the United States annually.[16] About four hundred thousand pacemakers are now placed in the United States every year. Millions of Americans live with an implanted pacemaker.[17]

It Will Help . . . It May Help . . . Or Maybe Not

The American College of Cardiology sets guidelines for the conditions in which pacemakers are beneficial. The ACC categorizes these conditions into situations where pacemakers are

1. Recommended (there is a strong reason to place a pacemaker)
2. Reasonable (there is good enough reason to place a pacemaker) or
3. Not unreasonable (there is a very weak reason to place a pacemaker).

In 1984, the ACC suggested fifty-six conditions for which pacemakers were either *recommended* or considered *reasonable*. By 2008, this number had grown to eighty-eight. The majority of the newer conditions for placing a pacemaker fell under the "reasonable" or "not unreasonable" categories. Unfortunately, only 5 percent of these guidelines are based on clinical trials, the overwhelming majority of them based on either expert opinions or standard of care in absence of scientific evidence.[18]

With the increased ease of the procedures, a growing number of disease states where it is "not unreasonable" to place pacemakers along with good rates of reimbursement have resulted in an increasing number of physicians becoming comfortable with recommending them easily. At some point, however, this comfort has given way to unscrupulous use.

In the past, doctors would have carefully examined whether there was an absolute benefit to the patient to be derived from the pacemakers or not, but over time doctors began to look at borderline cases or gray zones and say, "Well, I have enough here to justify it, so I'm going to do it."[19] In other words, it is "not unreasonable" for them to place a pacemaker, so they proceed with it. Patients who in the past would have undergone vigorous evaluation prior to getting pacemakers now get them because the doctor can justify putting it rather than because they know the patient will benefit from it.

Generally placing pacemakers in a patient with a specific condition could be justified and considered "not unreasonable" per ACC guidelines (see figure 6.1).

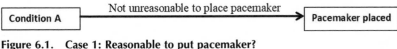

Figure 6.1.   Case 1: Reasonable to put pacemaker?
Author

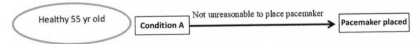

Figure 6.2. Case 2: Reasonable to put pacemaker?
Author

For example, an otherwise healthy fifty-five-year-old who is passing out because of slow heart rate will benefit from a pacemaker (see figure 6.2).

However, in truth, in the majority of patients having pacemakers placed do not have one specific disease but, rather, suffer from more than one severe or chronic condition. In those patients, though a pacemaker *can* be justified because they have one condition in which the pacemaker is *not unreasonable*, the pacemaker may not be beneficial to the patient because they have many other health issues. Many cases fall under this category where it becomes *unreasonable* to place a pacemaker if you take the complete situation into account (see figure 6.3).

In the 1990s, one in five patients received a pacemaker in the final year of their lives.[20] These patients had multiple chronic diseases, and though a pacemaker may have been justified for the one condition, in the presence of multiple conditions, it did not help. Pacemakers placed under these circumstances did nothing to increase the life span of these patients.

This problem of indiscriminate use was recognized as early as the 1980s. When the medical records of 382 pacemaker patients in Philadelphia County were reviewed in 1983, less than half of these cases had a well-documented need for the pacemaker. In this study it appeared that *one in five* patients received a pacemaker that they *did not need*.[21] Many other assessments conducted throughout the 1980s and 1990s showed that as many as *one in three* pacemaker implants were *not necessary*.[22] Furthermore, a study conducted by the Mayo Clinic found that when infected devices were removed from patients, *one in three* cases *did not* require a replacement: they had not needed the initial device in the first place.[23]

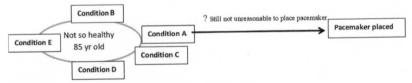

Figure 6.3. Case 3: Reasonable to put pacemaker?
Author

Certain recent cases of pacemaker placement abuse have been so blatant that the authorities had to intervene. In April 2018, the US Department of Justice successfully brought a case against cardiologist Dr. Anis Chalhoub after he placed about 234 pacemakers between 2007 and 2011.[24] Prosecutors were able to clearly show that dozens of those placements had been medically unnecessary, and a number of patients testified to being pressured into getting the pacemaker "to save your life" even when—as in Patricia's case—they merely had the nonfatal condition of a slow heart rate. This is an extreme case but one that shows the potential scale of the unnecessary placement of pacemakers if the practice continues.

All of these patients who receive these unnecessary pacemakers are subjected to fatal and nonfatal complications of pacemaker surgery. These include bleeding, infection, puncture of the heart, or collapse of the lungs during the surgery but also the possibility of infection of the pacemaker in the long run, possibility of blocked veins, a malfunctioning device, and so on.[25] Thankfully, Patricia did not suffer from any of these negative effects.

The Best Therapy for Patricia

In the weeks following Patricia's pacemaker surgery, Dr. Saleh performed a few tests and evaluations. After detailed assessment, taking all her symptoms into consideration, and ruling out other diseases, Patricia was diagnosed with the early stages of dementia. The diagnosis explained her forgetfulness, fatigue, and lack of interest in her favorite activities. She was started on the appropriate medications to slow down the progress of the disease.

The best therapy for her, Dr. Saleh suggested, was to move in with family to ensure her safety, keep her mentally engaged, and slow down the progression of the disease. Carla and her husband happily volunteered to have Patricia move in with them, and the benefit that she received from being around her loved ones was far greater than the pacemaker ticking inside her.

APPENDIX

What Is the Normal Electrical System of the Heart?

The heart has its own electrical system. The heart's spark plug is the *sinoatrial node*. The *SA node*, as it's known, located in the right upper chamber of the heart, starts a normal heartbeat. From here, the electrical activity spreads to the two upper chambers. The electricity then passes to the *atrioventricular junction*—or the *AV junction*—located between the upper and lower chambers. After a minor delay, the electricity spreads from the AV junction to the lower chamber, and contraction of these heart chambers follows the electrical signal. In a normal heart, the upper chambers get the electrical signal and contract first. Moments later, the lower chamber receives the electrical impulses and contracts in a rhythmic, coordinated manner (see figure 6.4).

Our brain and body require fifty to one hundred beats of the heart per minute to be properly supplied with oxygenated blood, though a rare group of very athletic people requires fewer beats when they are resting. A normal heart produces enough electrical activity in the SA node to meet the requirements of the body. Each of these beats then passes to the lower chamber.

Under certain circumstances, fewer than required beats are produced. This happens when either

1. The SA node slows down and produces an inadequate number of heart-beats or
2. The AV junction between the upper and lower chamber is damaged and so is not able to send each beat from the upper chamber down to the lower chamber.

How Do I Know If My Heart Is Not Producing Enough Beats?

If your heart beats too slowly, not enough blood flows through your body. This can cause

- Fatigue
- Fainting
- Shortness of breath
- A decrease in exercise capacity
- Increasing naps and
- Confusion.[26]

What Is a Pacemaker? How Does It work?

A *permanent pacemaker* (artificial pacemaker) has two parts:

1. The *pulse generator* is a small metal container containing a battery and the electrical circuitry. It sits underneath the skin next to your left or right shoulder and controls the electrical activity of the heart. Sometimes this is referred to as a *pacemaker* or as a *battery*.

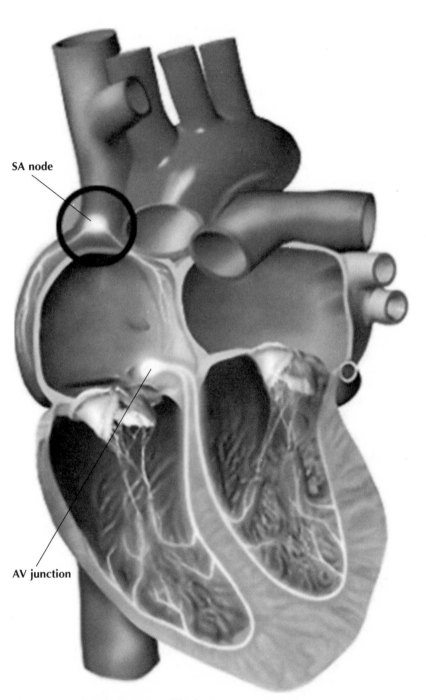

SA node

AV junction

Figure 6.4. Electrical system of the heart
Bruce Blaus

2. The *leads* (or *electrodes*) are wires that travel from the pulse generator to the heart. These wires connect the heart to the electrical circuitry in the pulse generator. Each heartbeat is monitored via these leads. If the beats are lower than required, the electrical signal will be sent from the battery to the heart via these leads.[27]

When there is a beat generated by the heart, the signal is picked up by the lead and travels to the pulse generator. The electrical circuitry registers it and waits for the next signal. If there is another signal, it waits for the one after that. If the next signal does not arrive on time, the electrical circuitry sends a signal to the lead, which transmits it to the heart muscle. This makes the heart beat. Thus pacemakers work in sync with the hearts own beats and provides beats only when required.

Most pacemakers have sensors. These detect your body motion and breathing rate and signal for the pacemaker to increase your heart rate during exercise. This will ensure that your body gets increased blood and oxygen for the duration of increased activity.

If My Heart Rate or Pulse Is Slow, Does That Mean I Need a Pacemaker?

In medicine, the same medical condition can be caused due to myriad different causes. As such, your heart rate may be slow for many reasons that do not require a pacemaker. These conditions include

- Taking medication that slows down the heart rate
- Thyroid-related problems
- Electrolyte problems
- Recent heart surgery
- Lifelong significant aerobic activities and
- Slower heart rate at night.[28]

In these situations, a pacemaker may not be required. If a patient has no symptoms related to slow heart rate, a pacemaker is generally not needed. Unlike in Patricia's case, before any treatment is decided upon, your personal heart rate record and general health *must* be taken into account. Think of health care as a jigsaw puzzle: You and your individual circumstances are always the final piece needed to complete it.

An exception is when there are normal heartbeats in a patient's upper chamber but a very low heart rate in the lower chamber due to disease in the AV junction (between the upper and lower chambers). Here a pacemaker is recommended even when there may be minimal symptoms.

What Are the Risks of the Pacemaker-Placement Procedure?

There are occasional complications that can occur while putting in a pacemaker, including

- Bruising or bleeding at the pacemaker site
- A collapsed lung
- Allergic reaction to the dye used
- Negative effects of the anesthesia used and
- Infection around the pacemaker site.

Over the long term, about one in ten patients experiences problems related to their pacemaker. Life-threatening complications of pacemaker implantation are rare.[29]

How Long Is the Hospital Stay after Pacemaker Placement?

At the time of the initial pacemaker placement, you will likely be required to stay in the hospital overnight. The next morning, you will get a chest X-ray, and someone will check the pacemaker using a laptop-like machine called a *programmer*. These tests make sure that the pacemaker leads are well positioned and working well.

How Will My Life Change after Getting a Pacemaker?

In the first week or two, you will be asked to **not**

- Lift your arm above the shoulder and
- Lift more than ten to fifteen pounds.

On a long-term basis, you may be asked to

- Avoid placing your cell phone directly over your pacemaker
- Avoid lingering near or leaning against a metal-detection system at the airport
- Carry an ID card to show that you have a pacemaker so that security personnel at the airport or other places where metal detection is used will carry out appropriate security checks on you without damaging your pacemaker
- Stand more than two feet away from welding equipment, high-voltage transformers, or motor-generator systems at all times

- Inform your team you have a pacemaker before undergoing any medical procedures, including MRI or surgeries
- Place a hospital-provided monitor next to your bed so the pacemaker can communicate with your physician's office and
- Come in for office visits every three to six months to get your device checked.

Devices like microwave ovens, televisions, remote controls, radios, toasters, electric blankets, electric shavers, electric drills, and other household electrical goods do not interfere with a pacemaker.

How Long Does the Pacemaker's Battery Last?

After the initial placement of the pacemaker, the battery will last five to twelve years. During your routine pacemaker checkup, its battery life will be checked. You will be informed when your battery has worn out and needs replacement. At that time, the pulse generator will be replaced with a new one, but the leads from the initial pacemaker will be retained. The changing-out of the battery is a much simpler procedure than the initial placement. The recovery is also quicker, and there are fewer precautions.[30]

Are There Different Types of Pacemakers?

Depending on the number of wires going into the heart, pacemakers can be

- *Single chamber*, with one wire going to the right lower chamber or, on rare occasions, with the single wire placed in the right upper chamber instead
- *Dual chamber*, with two wires, one going to the right upper chamber and another to the right lower chamber, or
- *Biventricular*, which consists of three wires, one going to the right upper chamber, another to right lower chamber, and the third to the left lower chamber.

What Questions Should I Ask My Physician before Signing Up for the Procedure?

- Why do I need a pacemaker?
- Could my condition be temporary?
- Could the condition be reversed without a pacemaker?
- What happens if I do not get a pacemaker?
- What improvement will I notice after a pacemaker?

- Will I get a single, dual, or biventricular pacemaker?
- What happens if I wait to decide on whether I want a pacemaker or not?
- Is the pacemaker going to be MRI-compatible?
- Is the pacemaker going to be monitored from home?
- Do you have a device clinic to monitor my device regularly?

7

Defibrillator: Many Get It, Some Need It

Temporary solutions often become permanent problems.

—Craig Bruce[1]

ICD
AKA: INTERNAL CARDIOVERTER-DEFIBRILLATOR

A Perfect Life Takes a Turn

It was funny how the congratulations and consolations came back-to-back for Jessica.

Jessica and Josh had been together for about two years before he'd proposed. Within three months, they were married, and soon she was pregnant with their first child—the first of three, they planned. They bought their first house shortly afterward—a four-bedroom ranch-style home with a large backyard, big enough for the family they anticipated. The couple was blissfully happy, pleased that things were falling into place quickly.

Jessica's pregnancy progressed without a hitch, aside from some back pain she suffered in the later stages. However, even this was bearable because the pain served as a reminder of the baby's impending arrival.

Jordan Elizabeth Douglas was born on January 9, 2010. She was 7.5 pounds, twenty inches long, and instantly became the center of their lives. Like all new parents, they ignored their own needs to ensure the comfort of the baby, so when Jessica started coughing, she thought nothing of it. It was probably some viral infection that would pass soon, she figured. She dreaded the idea of letting Jordan out of her sight even for the duration of a short visit to the doctor. However, the cough kept getting worse, and soon she was getting out of breath. She surrendered to her body's needs and called the doctor's office. Thankfully, they had a same-day opening.

Phoebe, the physician's assistant, was there to greet Jessica when she arrived. Prior to the examination, she agreed with Jessica that it was likely to be something viral, but surprisingly, when she listened to Jessica's lungs, something didn't seem right.

Phoebe ordered an urgent chest X-ray, which confirmed that Jessica's heart was enlarged and there was fluid in her lungs. Instead of the anticipated antibiotics or cough syrup, Jessica walked out with water pills to get rid of the fluid in her lungs, and Phoebe scheduled her for an echocardiogram appointment.

"It's an ultrasound of the heart, just to check if your heart muscles are pumping normally," she had explained.

The water pills had an instant impact. Within a couple of days, Jessica's cough was gone and she was breathing better. She wondered if she still needed the echocardiogram and called to ask Phoebe about it.

Phoebe sounded confident. "You had fluid in the lungs, which may be due to a weak heart muscle. I would like to make certain that your heart is working well."

Jessica trusted that Phoebe was acting in her best interest. Reluctantly, she took some more time away from Jordan for the echocardiogram. It would only be a quick thirty-minute visit.

Before the procedure, Jessica asked the technician if the echocardiogram would be like those ultrasounds they used to do on her belly while she was pregnant.

"Yep, it's exactly like that," the technician explained, "except instead of looking at the baby, we look at the heart. Sadly, it's not as cute!"

* * *

The next day, Phoebe called to inform Jessica that her heart was indeed weak, pumping at a mere 30 percent. Phoebe added that she had made a referral, and Jessica was to follow up with a cardiologist. Jessica was dumbfounded; how could this be? She had always eaten right, even as a teenager. She had never smoked a day in her life and ran three or four days a week.

She called her parents, and they were just as shocked. Only two weeks before, they had been congratulating her on the birth of her baby, and now she had a heart condition! They consoled her that maybe it had been a mistake; perhaps somebody else's echocardiogram had been confused with hers.

"These medical errors happen all the time. They even operate on the wrong patients. I've read about it in the newspapers," her father had said. "Let's wait to get to the specialist to sort this out."

The appointment with the cardiologist could not come soon enough for any of them. Jessica's parents agreed to accompany her to see Dr. Shankman, who had saved their neighbor's life.

Big Words, Big Worries

"This is a clear case of peripartum cardiomyopathy, which is a weakness of the heart after delivery. We can try some medication to see if it helps; some patients do recover, and their heart improves," Dr. Shankman summarized.

"Jessica is young, so there's a good chance of recovery, right?" her mother asked.

"We cannot predict which patients will improve, but let's hope you're right."

The doctor's words rang hollow in Jessica's ears. "What if I don't?" she asked, dejectedly.

"Let's cross that bridge when we come to it," Dr. Shankman said calmly. "Take the medicine regularly, and we'll see what happens."

The family was distraught, stunned into silence. They left the clinic and picked up the prescribed medicines.

Over the next few days, Jessica felt better, and her strength returned. When she and Josh went for a follow-up cardiology appointment two weeks later, they were optimistic that everything would be back to normal and were keen to put the nightmare behind them. The echocardiogram was repeated, and Dr. Shankman met with them again.

"Unfortunately, there has not been much change in your echocardiogram. The heart muscles continue to be weak, despite the medication. You're at risk for sudden cardiac death due to fatal heart-rhythm problems; I think we should schedule you for a defibrillator insertion." He said all of this matter-of-factly.

The couple was dazed, feeling as though they had been thrown into a stormy ocean and were struggling against huge waves.

Dr. Shankman explained that the defibrillator was a machine like a pacemaker, with wires inside the heart to detect fatal heart rhythms and shock the patient out of them, saving their life. "It's like insurance against sudden cardiac death. It will make sure that you see this young one grow up and go to college one day," he concluded, gesturing to Jordan.

What with how well she was feeling, Jessica had entertained high hopes that her heart muscles were recovering. Instead, she was returning home with terrifying terms swirling around her mind—*sudden cardiac death . . . defibrillator . . . fatal heart rhythm*. Along with Josh, she was trying to make sense of this situation, but she felt like she was drowning.

The next day, Dr. Shankman's nurse called to schedule the defibrillator placement. She repeated his words: "This will be like an insurance policy against a rhythm problem. Not everyone in your condition has fatal arrhythmia. However, if you do, the defibrillator will save your life. I always say it's better to have a defibrillator and not need to use it to save you from fatal heart rhythm than to need it because you have a fatal heart rhythm and *not* have it."

Jessica felt that her fate was unfair. She had done everything right, and yet she was still having heart problems at such a young age. However, as Josh had said, having this procedure was a no-brainer. She had to go ahead and get this defibrillator for herself and her family. But she felt so lost! It felt as if a train were hurtling toward her at unrelenting speed, and she had little strength to get out of its path. But who could argue with taking every measure to avoid sudden death?

She was very grateful when the nurse offered her a spot on the schedule the following week. The anxiety that had taken over her family would be mollified once she got this defibrillator. It would apparently act like a bulletproof vest to protect against all ills of the heart.

But how had developments in science and technology managed to create such a device anyway?

One Good Invention Deserves Another

In the mid-1900s, progress in engineering had led to the invention of electronic heart monitors, which had made it possible to continuously monitor the heart rhythm of cardiac patients. It soon became clear that an abnormal heart rhythm from the lower chambers of the heart—the *ventricles*—was an important cause of cardiac death.

When a heart goes into this type of rhythm—into *ventricular tachycardia, VT*, or *ventricular fibrillation, VF*—the instant delivery of large electrical shocks could restore normal rhythm and save the patient's life. The external defibrillator—invented by Dr. Bernard Lown in 1962—was a device capable of delivering such an electric shock.[2] These external defibrillators soon became the cornerstone of intensive-care units across the Western world, saving the lives of hundreds of cardiac patients every year.

However, hundreds of thousands more were still dying at home, when not under the supervision of a physician. It was a true public-health problem in the Western world. How could fatal rhythms that occurred at home be treated?

It would take the foresight, genius, and perseverance of a Polish immigrant to solve this conundrum.

In 1924, Michel Mirowski was born into a comfortably middle-class Jewish family that was part of the vibrant Jewish community in Warsaw during the 1920s and 1930s. But when Nazi Germany invaded Poland, Michel, only fifteen years old, saw the approaching danger and fled to Russia with a friend. While the war raged on, he managed to evade German troops, Russian authorities, and even starvation. He was the only person in his family to survive the Second World War.

After the war, he briefly returned to Poland, where he started medical school. Soon after, he moved to Lyon, France, to complete his education, though he spoke little French. Having lived through the suffering and privations of war, attending medical school taught in an unfamiliar language could only constitute a minor annoyance.

Michel successfully graduated medical school and then further specialized in cardiology, working with respected cardiologists all across the globe—in Tel Aviv, Mexico City, Baltimore, and Staten Island. He eventually returned to Tel Aviv for his first job, where he discovered that his supervisor suffered frequent bouts of abnormal heart rhythm, frequently passing out from it at home as well as at work. The man soon succumbed to his VT, and Michel's interest in better treating patients suffering dangerous arrhythmias was kindled. He determined to invent a device that would help save lives. The prototype he envisioned would function like the external defibrillator, giving patients a large enough shock to treat their VT or VF, but it would be placed *inside* the patient's body, where its life-saving shocks could be automated, working all on its own without human intervention. In effect, Michel wanted to create the first *internal defibrillator*.[3]

Against All Odds

Michel got the opportunity to realize his idea in 1968, when he was recruited to head the coronary unit at Sinai Hospital of Baltimore. There he met Morton Mower, a young colleague who shared Michel's passion and vision for the development of the internal defibrillator or *implantable cardioverter-defibrillator (ICD)* as it would be called. Working with the biomedical engineering department, they formed the ideal team.[4]

After significant effort, they successfully created a prototype, proving its effectiveness in a dog in 1969. They published their work but faced heavy criticism from many cardiologists of the time. In 1972, Dr. Lown, inventor of the external defibrillator, stated in a journal that "the implanted defibrillator system *represents an imperfect solution in search of a plausible and practical application*."[5] Such criticism could have been the kiss of death for any invention.

However, Michel and Morton persevered. They were fortunate enough to meet Stephen Heilman, a physician, engineer, and entrepreneur, who shared their vision. He showed immense interest in their work, providing substantial resources to expand the team and develop the ICD further. Within three years, the team had produced another ICD prototype, this one small enough to be implanted within a dog. In 1975, they filmed a dog being successfully treated with the implanted ICD. The video sent shockwaves through the medical community and marked the official entry of the ICD into the arsenal of cardiac interventions.

Birth of a Lifesaver

Over the next five years, the group continued to evolve their invention, refining it for implantation in humans. Their efforts paid off, and in February 1980, along with colleagues at Johns Hopkins Hospital, they performed the first implant of an ICD into a human. The initial version had to be implanted by a surgeon after opening up the chest, but as time went on, Michel and Morton continued to miniaturize the ICD. By the late 1980s, they had succeeded in developing a model that could be placed through a small incision in the skin. This, among other changes, ensured that a cardiologist could now place the ICD instead of requiring the aid of a surgeon.[6]

Great Technology, but Who Needs It?

It was a well-known fact that like Michel's previous supervisor, patients who had once been revived from a fatal heart rhythm (a VT or VF) would invariably suffer repeat episodes. Therefore, the initial use of the ICD was tested on patients who had previously been revived. A research trial was undertaken to prove the effectiveness of the ICD compared to the available medicines.

New technologies always face their share of skeptics, and medical technologies more than others. Many cardiologists were sure that medication could do a better job treating arrhythmias than could this new, unknown device. They did not want their patients in the research trials testing the effectiveness of the ICD. However, thanks to a few visionary cardiologists, the research trials progressed. Within eighteen months, there was a clear winner: Patients with ICD were living longer than those without. For every four patients who had an ICD, one life was saved! The impact of the ICD was very obvious. The research testing was terminated, and ICDs were recommended for all those who had been revived from VT or VF.[7]

The skeptics had finally had a change of heart! ICDs, once written off as "an imperfect solution in search of a plausible and practical application," were now considered a lifesaver.

Patients who had survived their first instance of VT or VF could get an ICD implanted before their second episode. However, many never made it to the hospital alive after their first event, and attention quickly turned to these patients. Was there a way to identify people who were at higher risk of VT or VF? Could a preemptively placed ICD help them?

Saving Even More Lives

In the late 1990s and 2000s, attention shifted to patients at risk for VT or VF and on the prevention of death from their very first episode. Patients who despite medication continued to have weak hearts—*cardiomyopathy*—were considered to be at high risk for VT or VF. And so scientists studied the effect of preemptively placed ICDs in these patients. The initial focus was on people who had cardiomyopathy related to heart attacks, but as time passed, patients who suffered with cardiomyopathy regardless of the reason were studied. All of these studies were a big success, and the preemptive placement of an ICD saved the lives of many patients with a persistently weak heart muscle.[8] The professional cardiology societies officially endorsed preemptive placement of ICDs.[9]

Smooth Sailing

Jessica had her ICD placed. The procedure went smoothly, and she was discharged the next day. She experienced minor pain at the site of the surgery for about three days. She met up with the nurse the next week and found that the ICD was working well. Soon, she was feeling healthy again.

The day Jordan turned two months old, Jessica had yet another echocardiogram and visit with Dr. Shankman.

After receiving the test results, the doctor walked in beaming. "Hello, Jessica! Do you want the good news first or the good news first?" he joked. This was the first time she had seen him smile in all her visits. "Your heart muscles have recovered fully. The heart is pumping normally now."

Wow, back to normal! Jessica was thrilled that the nightmare was over. She felt like a kid who has just received an A+ on her finals! Her diligence with the medication and her careful diet and exercise regime had paid off. She couldn't wait to leave the doctor's office to call Josh and give him the good news; Jordan's two-month birthday celebration suddenly got a whole lot sweeter!

A Shocking Development

Four years later, Jessica was well and truly back to her routine. Other than the ICD near her left shoulder, she showed little sign of her previous heart troubles. Jordan was growing stronger and faster by the minute and wanted to play all day long. While chasing her around the backyard one day, out of the blue Jessica felt a thud in her chest. She doubled over in agony; it felt like a horse had kicked her. Before she could recover, she felt another shock, and within two minutes, there was a third. She yelled for Josh. Josh rushed to her and helplessly watched her reel from the shocks before racing to call 911. By the time EMS had arrived, Jessica had received fourteen shocks from the ICD and was in tears of anguish.

The EMTs transported her to the emergency room, where they stopped further shocks. Within an hour, the device technician came over and checked the ICD using a special laptop. She confirmed the fourteen shocks that Jessica had received in a nonchalant manner: "Yes, you had inappropriate shocks."

Jessica was in a daze and could not respond, but Josh entered the room moments later.

Once he had introduced himself, the technician repeated, "She had inappropriate shocks."

"*Inappropriate*? What do you mean? Dr. Shankman told us that the ICD would shock when her heart went into a fatal rhythm . . . VT, I think. Isn't that what happened?"

"No, there was no VT or VF. The device misdiagnosed it, which happens occasionally. Sometimes the ICD shocks even when the shocks are not needed. Therefore, they call it *inappropriate shock*."

The technician made air quotes casually, and Josh wondered angrily if she had any idea what Jessica was going through.

Seemingly unaware of his frustration, the technician continued. "In your wife's particular case, one of the wires of the ICD appears to be fractured. The ICD misdiagnosed the normal heartbeat as VF and gave her the shocks. Dr. Shankman will talk to you about replacing the wire with another one."

Quiet until now, Jessica broke down at the thought of another surgery, while Josh did his best to console her. She was admitted to the hospital, where both of them spent a sleepless night. Jessica kept thinking about the excruciatingly painful shocks and the possibility of their returning, while Josh worried about his wife and daughter and what impact all this may have on their family.

Thankfully, Dr. Shankman visited them first thing in the morning.

"It seems the wire is broken, so the ICD is diagnosing a normal rhythm as VF and then shocking you to treat it," he said. "Let me pull up the X-ray so you can see," showing them the chest X-ray that had been performed in the ER the night before. "You see this wire down here? It is intact all along, except—" he pointed the tip of his pen to the part of the wire closest to her shoulder"—right here, it appears broken."

Jessica and Josh could see a kink in the wire at that spot on the X-ray.

"The shocks you got yesterday," continued Dr. Shankman, "were inappropriate and were due to this fractured wire. To avoid further shocks, that broken wire needs to be replaced."

"When can we do that?" asked Jessica, eager to get the fractured wire out before it brought on more shocks.

"Well," hedged the doctor, "it's a little more complicated than putting it in the first time was. The wire has become part of your body and is enmeshed with your heart muscle. As a result, there are risks in bringing out the wire, because part of your heart tissue could break loose." His words were not reassuring.

"But it will all work out fine, right?" Josh realized that Jessica needed some positive talk rather than yet another issue to worry about.

There was a pause before the doctor nodded and continued. "We don't do that procedure here. I'll call the folks at University and transfer you under their care. It's best that you have the procedure done out there."

"Why the University Hospital? Is it a risky procedure? What can go wrong?" Jessica was already thinking of the worst-case scenario.

"It's a little risky, and there are always chances of complication. It's better to have it done at University. They can do it more safely there."

None of this was soothing Jessica's angst. She did not want to deal with any of this and felt like running away and returning to Jordan. But then she thought of those shocks. Once again, she felt that she had no choice. She had to go through with the next procedure.

*   *   *

The next day, Jessica was transferred to the University Hospital. The doctors there agreed that the wire was fractured and needed changing. Once again, the procedure went smoothly, and she was discharged to go home. The next week, Jessica had the device checked at Dr. Shankman's office.

All was well with the device, but Jessica was still distraught. She continued to think about the shocks from the ICD and struggled to sleep. When she did finally nod off, she would wake up drenched in sweat, having had a nightmare of getting shocked by the ICD again.

Seeking medical help for the anxiety that was now permeating her life, she was soon diagnosed with PTSD from the shocks and spent the next two years under the care of a psychologist before she could begin to get back to feeling normal.

Was Jessica just unfortunate, or is this a common occurrence?

A Rare Case . . . Or Is It?

The evidence and endorsements for the use of ICDs mounted throughout the late 1990s and early 2000s.[10] The benefit of ICDs and the ease of the procedure resulted in widespread acceptance of this technology among cardiologists. Since the FDA approved the first ICD in 1985, the number of ICDs placed in the United States has soared to over half a million total placements, and between 2005 and 2010 more than seventy thousand lives were saved by ICDs.[11] Medicare and other insurance plans compensate very well for an ICD implant, as the procedure itself costs about thirty-five thousand dollars.

As a result, the ICD has rapidly become one the most expensive medical devices in current use. The combination of its proven efficacy, the ease of its implantation, and its lucrative reimbursement has ensured an ever-increasing number of device implantations year on year.[12]

However, in a landmark study, researchers looked into the pattern of ICD implants around the country. In the three-year period between 2006 and 2009, they estimate that a little over one in five ICDs placed were unnecessary.[13] Other studies validate these findings.[14] In other words, thousands of patients who would not benefit from an ICD were nevertheless fitted with one.

Which Patients Received ICDs They Didn't Need?

Patients with an initial diagnosis of weak heart muscles (cardiomyopathy) need to be treated with medication. If after a *ninety-day* course of treatment there is no recovery, the patient needs an ICD. If the heart function improves, an ICD is not needed.[15] While this is clearly stated in the guidelines offered by all professional societies, physicians seem to rush to place ICDs without giving enough time for medication to work—as happened in Jessica's case. As a result, *one in five patients have received an ICD they did not need.*[16]

Another group that may not benefit from ICDs is older patients. ICDs prevent a significant number of deaths in younger people—below the age of seventy—when placed for the right reasons. However, among older patients and those with other noncardiac diseases, the benefit of ICDs is questionable. Older patients die frequently as a result of other causes, including cancer and pneumonia, which ICDs do not help. Therefore, these older patients succumb to these other noncardiac conditions and do not enjoy an increase in their life span despite the implantation of ICDs.[17]

In health care as in life, it is common for *action bias* to sneak in. This type of bias is based on the natural human tendency to take charge and act. A classic example of action bias is a soccer goalkeeper who jumps to grab the ball when facing a penalty kick even though it is well known in the soccer world that they will be more likely to intercept the ball and prevent a goal if they stay near the center of the net.[18] Have you ever had a desire to detour from your standard route to work and take a longer way just to prevent sitting in traffic? If so, that is your action bias—your desire to act even when you are uncertain that your action will actually help. Physicians are go-getters by nature and by training; they are taught to intervene and act to save lives. This tendency to be proactive takes over even when the research on whether action is better than restrained observation is unclear. Their subconscious action bias often makes physicians act sooner rather than wait. It is possible that this tendency to act may also lead physicians to implant ICDs early on in the course of the disease rather than wait to see if the condition will resolve itself naturally.

But What's the Harm?

Among those patients who received an ICD unnecessarily, rates of complication and death were three times higher than in those who actually needed it. Based on the number of ICDs placed, it has been estimated that one hundred more deaths have occurred because of faults in these devices than would have occurred without them. It appears that the same physicians implanting ICDs indiscriminately also happen to be poor at performing the implanting procedure and cause more complications.[19]

Besides the issue of determining correct or incorrect use, the devices are not perfect. Among all those who receive ICDs, one out of every five also receive an "inappropriate shock" like Jessica did. These are shocks that are given automatically by the ICD even when the patient does not have any abnormal rhythm. All shocks, whether appropriate or inappropriate, can damage the heart in the long run. As a result, patients who receive inappropriate shocks suffer a decrease in life span.[20] Furthermore, these ICD shocks can make patients anxious or depressed, and like Jessica, some of them suffer from PTSD.[21]

Just as with pacemaker implantation, ICD implantation carries the risk of infection, bleeding, and puncture of the heart or lungs during the procedure. And there are long-term risks of infection related to the ICD.[22]

In conclusion, therefore, among patients who do not need them, the "treatment" of ICD implantation is inherently worse than the disease itself.

There have also been several instances of flawed devices harming patients.[23] The adverse effects caused by faulty devices have recently undercut the confidence in ICDs, especially because in certain instances it has come to light that companies knowingly sold defective ICDs. In January 2011, one ICD manufacturer, Guidant Corporation, agreed to pay a 296-million-dollar fine after pleading guilty to failing to report device problems to the FDA.[24]

Is Anyone Held Accountable for Unnecessary ICDs?

Josh was spending a lazy Sunday morning reading the newspaper on his tablet. Thanks to his previous searches, he was regularly receiving articles regarding news on ICDs. Today's headline drew his attention: "Nearly 500 Hospitals Pay United States More Than $250 Million to Resolve False Claims Act Allegations Related to Implantation of Cardiac Devices."[25]

The article explained that the Department of Justice had investigated ICD placement across several hospitals. In almost five hundred hospitals physicians had not complied with guidelines in deciding when to place ICDs. These guidelines suggest that after the diagnosis of a weak heart muscle, patients needed to be treated with medication for a minimum of ninety days. The guidelines also state that in many cases, the heart recovers within three months and no further treatment is required. The DOJ investigation had uncovered that physicians had failed to wait the required ninety days in an overwhelming number of cases before implanting devices.

The article provided a long list of hospitals that had settled with the Department of Justice for misusing these ICD implants. The fines ran into the millions of dollars.

Josh's heart skipped a beat. He went to the master-bedroom closet and pulled out the copy of Jessica's medical file. He rechecked the papers and the dates, counting out the days between diagnosis, treatment, and the normalization of her heart function. Jessica's ICD had been placed within thirty days of the treatment, and she had fully recovered within sixty days of the treatment with medication. He could not believe it—if their doctor had waited the required ninety-day period to test the medication, Jessica would not have needed the ICD! He went back to the article and looked up the list of hospitals. Sure enough, Jessica's hospital was indeed one of them!

* * *

Following legal intervention, the hospital settled Jessica's case with the federal agencies, without so much as a personal apology to Jessica. The family had changed the course of their life because of the ICD, settling with Jordan rather than the three kids they had planned, and Jessica had suffered through PTSD for two years. All the struggles and the angst over the diagnosis had been for nothing!

Josh wondered if he would ever trust the medical system again. He suspected that the fear of terms like *sudden death, fatal heart rhythm,* and *defibrillator* had made them rush into getting the ICD. The fear of death had pushed them into getting surgery without a moment's pause. He questioned whether it would have been better to gather more information before signing up for it.

Looking back, would a second opinion have prevented Jessica from getting the ICD and the host of issues that came with it?

Should he tell Jessica what he had found out about her ICD?

APPENDIX

What Is the Normal Electrical System of the Heart?

As we first learned in chapter 6, the heart has its own electrical system. Normal heartbeats start in the SA node, located in the right upper chamber. From here, the electrical activity spreads to the two upper chambers. The electricity then conducts to the junction between the upper and lower chambers. After a minor delay, it spreads to the lower chamber, and contraction of the heart chambers follows the electrical signal. In a normal heart, the upper chambers get the electrical signal and then contract, and within one-tenth of a second, the lower chamber gets electricity and contracts in a similarly rhythmic, coordinated manner (see figure 7.1).

What Are the Life-Threatening Rhythm Problems?

Under certain circumstances, a normal heart rhythm gets disrupted. As a result, patients can have an abnormal rhythm. *Most abnormal rhythms are harmless.* However, there can also be infrequent heart-rhythm problems arising from the lower chambers (ventricles). Erratic heart rhythms coming from the ventricles—called ventricular tachycardia (VT) or ventricular fibrillation (VF)—disrupt the normal pumping of the blood. This disruption stops the supply of blood and oxygen to the body. VT or VF can quickly become life-threatening and cause the person to collapse within seconds. This is an emergency that requires immediate medical attention and is the most frequent cause of sudden cardiac death. Emergency treatment includes *cardiopulmonary*

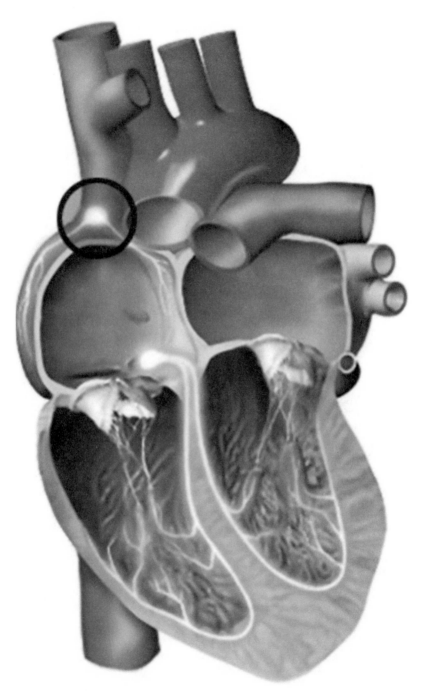

Figure 7.1. Electrical system of the heart
Bruce Blaus

resuscitation, better known as *CPR*, and shocks to the heart delivered by a device called an *automated external defibrillator*, or *AED*.

Who Gets Life-Threatening Arrhythmias?

VT or VF can occur within the first few hours and even days after a heart attack. In the long run, these two conditions commonly occur in patients who have weak hearts—a condition called *cardiomyopathy*. This weakness of the heart muscle can be due to several reasons:

- One or more heart attacks
- Untreated long-term high blood pressure
- Heart valve problems
- Long-term alcohol abuse
- Viral infection
- Cancer-related medication
- Drug abuse
- Postpregnancy and
- Certain cancer treatments.[26]

Are There Other Conditions that Can Cause Life-Threatening Rhythm Problems?

In short, yes. These can include

- Rare genetic conditions, such as Brugada syndrome or long QT syndrome
- Electrolyte imbalance and
- Congenital heart disease.[27]

How Will I Know If I Have Life-Threatening Heart-Rhythm Problems?

Ventricular tachycardia (VT) and ventricular fibrillation (VF) are life-threatening heart arrhythmias that can cause

- Chest pain
- Rapid heartbeat (*tachycardia*)
- Dizziness
- Nausea
- Shortness of breath and
- Loss of consciousness.[28]

How Are VT and VF Treated?

Instances of VT and VF are life-threatening emergencies. If you are with someone you suspect is experiencing VT or VF, based on the above symptoms, you *must*

- Call 911 (or the emergency number where you are)
- Check for a pulse
- If there is no pulse, begin CPR: and
- Try to find a portable AED, which can deliver an electrical shock that may restore normal heart rhythm. AEDs are available in an increasing number of places, such as aboard airplanes, in police cars, or at shopping malls. Most of them come with built-in instructions for use and will only deliver a shock when needed.

The EMTs will then arrive and take over the care.

What Is an ICD? Defibrillator? Internal Defibrillator?

An *ICD* is a small device about the size of a pager or a pocket watch. It is surgically placed under the skin, typically close to the shoulder and below the left collarbone. One or more wires, called *leads*, run from the ICD through your veins to your heart.

The ICD can detect abnormal heart rhythms and instantly attempt to correct them by giving a shock to restore normal heart rhythm (see figure 7.2).[29]

Who Needs an ICD?

Patients who have been revived from fatal heart rhythm VT or VF have a greater chance of having another such incident. They are ideal candidates for an ICD.

Others who may require an ICD preemptively are

- Patients with a weak heart muscle (*cardiomyopathy*) with *ejection fraction*, or *EF*—a measure of the heart's pumping strength—of less than 35 percent (the normal range can go from 55 to 65 percent), despite using medication to improve it.
  - If the heart muscles are weak after a heart attack, it is recommended to wait for at least forty days before implanting an ICD.

Implantable Cardioverter Defibrillator

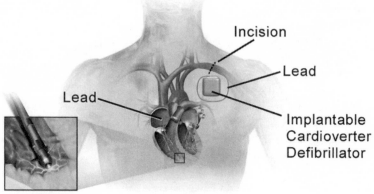

Incision

Lead

Lead

Implantable
Cardioverter
Defibrillator

Tip of lead in right
ventricle of Heart

Figure 7.2.   Implantable cardioverter-defibrillator
Bruce Blaus

○ If the heart muscles are weak due to any other reason, it is recommended to try medication for at least ninety days before implanting an ICD.
• Patients with a rare inherited heart disease, including long QT syndrome, Brugada syndrome, or arrhythmogenic right ventricular dysplasia.[30]

What Are the Risks of the ICD Procedure?

Risks associated with ICD implantation may include

• Infection at the site of the ICD implant
• Swelling, bleeding, or bruising where your ICD was implanted
• Bleeding around your heart, which can be life threatening
• Collapsed lung (*pneumothorax*)
• Allergic reaction to the medications used during the procedure and
• Clots forming in the vein where your ICD leads are placed.[31]

What Can I Expect after an ICD Is Placed?

You will get an appointment to check the surgical site one week after implantation. You will also have a monitor sitting by your bedside which automatically sends daily reports of any unusual events to the physician's office. You will be asked to come in, in person once or twice a year to get the ICD checked, and the ICD battery will need changing every five to seven years.

On average, out of one hundred patients receiving ICDs over a five-year period,

- Seven to eight patients will be shocked and saved by their ICD
- Ten to twenty will get a shock that they don't need
- Five to fifteen will have other complications
- Thirty will die whether or not they have an ICD because of a condition unrelated to the heart and
- Thirty-two will neither benefit from nor be harmed by the ICD.[32]

How Much Benefit Will I Get Out of an ICD Placement?

There have been various studies of patients with a heart attack and related weak heart muscle who get the ICD preemptively, before their first instance of abnormal heart rhythm. *For every eight patients getting the ICD, one life will be saved every three years.* This is considered a magnificent outcome, especially if you are the one!

In those who have a weak heart muscle but have not had a heart attack and who have an ICD placed, over a three-year period, *one out of twenty-five will have their life saved due to the device.*[33]

What Questions Should I Ask My Surgeon before Signing Up for the Procedure?

Why Are We Putting the ICD In?

See whether or not you fall under any of the above-specified categories.

What Kind of Benefit Can I Expect from the ICD?

ICDs are used to prevent sudden death related to heart rhythm. Patients who have been revived from one episode of fatal heart rhythm get the most benefit from ICD. For every four patients having ICDs under these circumstances, one life will be saved.

Patients who have weak heart pumping due to one or more heart attacks preemptively get an ICD. For every eight of these patients having an ICD for three years, one life is saved.

Patients who have weak heart pumping due to any other reason preemptively get an ICD after medication has failed to restore the pumping to normal. For every twenty-five patients in these circumstances who have had an ICD for three years, one life is saved.[34]

Is Having an ICD Going to Prolong My Life, Considering All My Other Diseases?

If you have cancer that is decreasing your life span or advanced lung disease or if you are of advanced age, the ICD may prevent heart-rhythm-related death. However, it will not prevent death due any other condition. In that case, an ICD may not prolong life.

If I Am Comfortable Passing Away in My Sleep or If I Do Not Want to Be Resuscitated, Would You Still Recommend an ICD?

This is an important question that is neither asked nor discussed enough. If you are eighty-five years old, have a poor quality of life for any reason—medical or otherwise—and are comfortable with the idea of passing away, a fatal VT or VF in the middle of the night is the ideal way to go. In that case, ICD is not a good option for you. However, if you are enjoying a good quality of life and believe that you would want to be revived from VT or VF, then an ICD should be considered.

A thorough discussion with family members and deliberation over this question is critical prior to undergoing an ICD implant.

What Are My Chances of Receiving an Inappropriate Shock from My ICD? How Can These Be Decreased?

Younger patients have a higher risk of inappropriate shocks because during exercise their heart rate can reach very high levels. Such a high heart rate can be misinterpreted as VT or VF by the ICD, and they can receive a resulting shock. Another group that can experience inappropriate shocks are patients with *atrial fibrillation* (a benign abnormal heart rhythm problem arising from the upper chambers of the heart). In atrial fibrillation, the lower chambers can pump at a faster rate and be misinterpreted as VT or VF by the ICD. If there is a problem with the ICD, such as a fracture of the wire, patients can get inappropriate shocks.

The first two conditions can be anticipated and the appropriate settings programmed in the ICD so that the chance of inappropriate shock decreases.

Am I at a Higher Risk than Average for Complications?

You are at higher risk of infection for ICD implantation if you

- Have diabetes
- Have cancer
- Are of increased age
- Take blood thinners
- Have frequent infections
- Have renal failure
- Have emphysema or COPD or
- Take medication to suppress your immune system, such as steroids.[35]

Infection risk is decreased by the use of intravenous antibiotics before the procedure.

What Is the Infection Rate in Your Lab?

The procedure room where your doctor is performing these surgeries, or the lab, should have an infection rate lower than 2 to 3 percent. Anything higher is too high to risk.

Are You an Electrophysiologist?

Electrophysiologists are popularly called "the electricians of the heart." They have additional training in taking care of heart-rhythm problems and an in-depth understanding of the need for ICDs. They have mastered the appropriate programming of ICDs so they can prevent inappropriate shocks by setting it correctly.

Will You Be the Physician Monitoring My ICD over the Long Term?

It is better to have a physician who is going to be your physician over the long run place the device.

Do You Think We Can Wait for My Heart Function to Improve So
That I Won't Need an ICD?

Patients who benefitted from their ICD had the life-saving shock in years two and three after the ICD implant. There is no rush for these devices, especially not when heart function can improve in some cases. If heart function improves, and the ejection fraction is greater than 35 percent, you may no longer benefit from an ICD. On the other hand, if you have an ICD fitted and then your heart function improves, the risk of removing the ICD is greater than the benefit. Physicians will not remove the ICD because your heart function has improved.

8

Ablation: Curing Your Rhythm Problems

Sometimes the smartest thing to do is nothing.

—Proverb

ABLATION
AKA: HEART ABLATION, CARDIAC ABLATION

If Only She Knew Then What She Knows Now

While sitting in her wheelchair in the doctor's waiting room, Corina listened to the Beatles on her iPhone. An eerie sense came over her when she heard Paul McCartney sing, "Yesterday, all my troubles seemed so far away . . ."

Dr. Susskind's nurse came out and started talking to the patients in the waiting area, as though she were making an announcement. By the time Corina had lifted her right hand to remove her earbuds, the nurse had finished her announcement, turned around, and left.

Corina turned to the person next to her—a healthy-looking woman who appeared to be in her late '60s, wearing a T-shirt that said *Ride, Sweat, Love* and a necklace strung from African beads. She reminded Corina of herself two years ago, and not just because she had a similar bicycling T-shirt and loved traveling.

"What did she say?" Corina asked. Her speech, garbled after the stroke, had improved a lot after a year of speech therapy.

"Dr. Susskind is running twenty minutes late." With a playful smile, the woman imitated the nurse broadly—"Sorry for the inconvenience."

Corina smiled back.

"How do you like that book?" the woman asked, pointing to the tome in Corina's lap titled *Cooked.*

"Oh, I'm not sure yet; I've just started reading it. Have you read it?" Corina was happy to be settling into a conversation; it seemed that they were going to be in the waiting room for a while.

"No, but a couple of colleagues at work were talking about it. I *have* read his previous book, *Omnivore's Dilemma.* That one turned me into a vegetarian."

"Yes, me too! I was so influenced by that book, I haven't eaten meat for ten years now." She turned her wheelchair to better face the woman. "And I don't even miss it anymore. It wasn't as difficult to cut it out as I thought it would be." Then she wryly noted, "But then again, it hasn't prevented us from having to visit the doctor, has it?"

"No, I guess broccoli won't prevent all that will ail you!" the other woman laughed, speaking for both of them.

There was a silence that stretched a few moments. It seemed maybe their natural small talk had met a dead end. But then the woman smiled again and turned to Corina.

"I'm Mary, by the way," she said, placing a hand on her chest.

"Hello, Mary. I'm Corina." Out of habit, she added, "Corina Stoudemire."

"Corina Stoudemire . . . like the CEO of Standard Oil?" Mary blurted, not bothering to weigh first whether it was polite to ask.

"Ha! I got found out! I don't *think* I'm a household name; how did you know?" Corina could not hide her pride.

"Well, in a city like Houston, oil executives rule," Mary explained. "Besides, I'm with Paragon Oil, so I'm kind of in the know."

"What do you do at Paragon, Mary? If you don't mind my asking, that is."

"I am their chief marketing officer."

Corina felt more familiar now that she knew they shared so much in common. "Well, you've got me curious. If you don't mind my asking, what do you see Dr. Susskind for?"

"A-fib," Mary replied. "Atrial fibrillation."

"Me too; I've had it for three years. How long have you had it?"

"It started about seven years ago. The frustrating part is, I don't have any other heart conditions. No other *health* conditions, as a matter of fact."

"Wow, that's so similar to my situation! I was happily going about my life, and out of the blue, boom! A-fib. Did you also find out about yours during an annual physical exam?" Corina probed further.

"No, I had some fluttering in the chest," Mary explained, "and they did a heart monitor and found out A-fib was causing this fluttering, or *palpitations*, as Dr. Susskind calls them."

"Do you still have it, or are you cured?"

"No, it still happens for eight to ten minutes once every two months or so. I come and see Dr. Susskind once a year for a wellness check, so to say," said Mary, smiling, with a shrug.

"But you're still having the A-fib. They're not going to fix it?"

"You mean with ablation?"

"Yes. I've had two, and I think I may need another one. I got fixed, and a year later, it came back. I had to undergo another one, and that was when . . ." Corina trailed off as the medical assistant came into the waiting room.

"Dr. Susskind is back. Mary, you're first; let's take you back."

As Mary rose, she turned toward Corina and extended her hand. "It was such a pleasure talking to you!"

"Same here. Good luck with the doctor's visit!"

Corina was disappointed that Mary had been called in for her appointment at that moment; she was curious to find out why Mary had not undergone ablation when both of them had the same disease and wished she could have had five more minutes with Mary to find out. Brow furrowed, she watched as Mary followed the assistant into the doctor's office.

A Mystery Problem

Debilitating heart-rhythm problems called *supraventricular tachycardia*, or *SVT* for short, impact the young as well as the old. As of the middle of the twentieth century, these heart-rhythm problems were known to be related to electrical problems of the heart that some unfortunate people simply had to bear. The mechanics of how SVTs originated was unknown. Certain medicines worked in about half of patients, but the other half received no apparent benefit. Though not life-threatening, episodes of SVTs greatly impacted some patients' quality of life as they suffered through spells of palpitations, lightheadedness, and, in some cases, fainting.

In the first step toward understanding the mechanics of these abnormal rhythm problems, medical pioneers in the 1940s and '50s began to better understand the heart's normal electrical activity when they placed metal electrodes at the tip of a catheter and passed it into a patient's heart through a big IV line in the groin. These electrodes made recordings of the electrical activity in different parts of the heart, effectively mapping the electrical progression as it sequenced through the heart.[1]

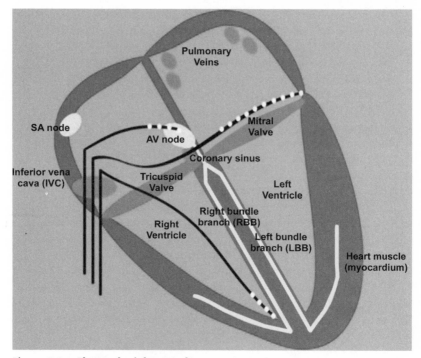

Figure 8.1.   Electrophysiology study
Nick Jackson

In 1958, scientists found a way to connect these electrode-tipped catheters to a stimulator and pass electricity inside the heart and induce heart signals. It was like applying a little spark of electricity within the heart, which provoked abnormal rhythm problems at will. Once the abnormal rhythm started, the catheters would record from various sites. Carefully measuring the time it took electricity to reach a certain electrode, they were able to map the path of the abnormal rhythm.[2]

These developments were crucial in understanding the mechanics of abnormal heart rhythms. It was recognized that the patients who suffered SVT episodes had an extra circuit in the heart. The extra circuit, though it measured mere millimeters, allowed short-circuiting of the heart rhythm and caused rapid, abnormal rhythms. The location of the extra circuit could be identified with precision by cardiologists using these electrode-tipped catheters. But after making the diagnosis and pinpointing the abnormal area in the heart, however, the cardiologist had to turn the patient over to the surgeon to operate on the trouble-making abnormal circuit. The surgeons would open up the patient's chest, cauterize this abnormal circuit, and cure the abnormal heart rhythm once and for all.

A Methodical Approach to Perfection

Cardiologists recognized that if they could load a cautery at the end of a catheter they can do themselves what the surgeons had been doing and cauterize the extra circuit. James Beazell, a researcher with Harbor-UCLA Medical Center had developed a technique wherein a direct current shock was provided at specific location in dogs via catheter. This destroyed some tissue just like a cautery would. It attracted the attention of prominent cardiologist Dr. Melvin Scheinman, who grew interested in replicating the procedure in humans. He recruited Chilean doctor Rolando Gonzalez to work with him on the project. The two made the trip to visit James Beazell to better understand his technique and then tried to replicate it on their own, forced to modify it further to achieve similar results. Scheinman confirmed that the technique was achieving permanent damage to the extra, malfunctioning circuit. Once convinced of the procedure's efficacy, he set out to try it in humans.

In 1981, at the University of San Francisco Medical Center, Melvin Scheinman and his team met the perfect patient: This man was quite impacted by his rhythm problem, so when surgeons had been asked to perform an open-heart surgery, they had declined, pointing out that the patient was too sick to undergo open heart procedure. And so the patient was between a rock and a hard place—sick enough to need immediate medical intervention but too fragile to risk the prevailing surgical treatment. Scheinman stepped in, offering to perform his new technique, explaining the team's success in dog models. Though the patient understood it had up until then been untested in humans, he agreed to undergo the procedure. The team placed a catheter in the man's heart and connected it to a direct current source. A shock was delivered to the tip of the catheter, damaging the tissue of the underlying area (see figure 8.2). Thus, using the small catheter passed through an IV line in the patient's groin, the team had performed the first *catheter ablation*, achieving what surgeons had only ever accomplished via open-heart surgery. The team had approached the issue systematically and succeeded in providing a stunning solution.[3]

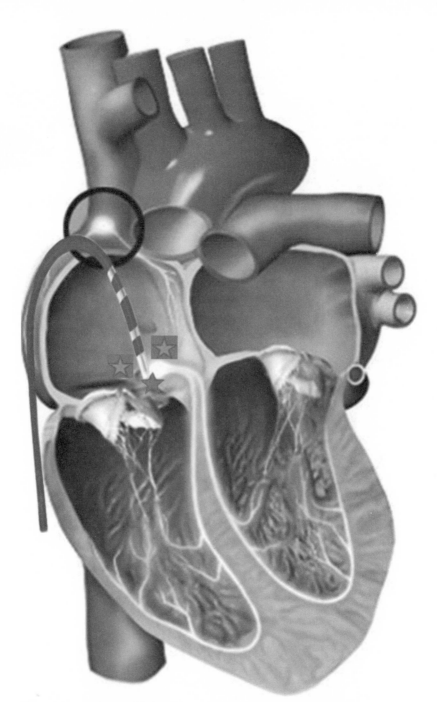

Figure 8.2.   Catheter ablation: Damaging a malfunctioning part of the heart using an electrode-tipped catheter

Modified from Bruce Blaus image

The Path to Perfection

Despite the team's enthusiasm at the discovery and the care with which it had evolved, their initial solution to use a direct current left a lot to be desired. The energy delivered caused cardiac rupture in some patients, as well as collateral damage in others. In certain other cases, the damage to the malfunctioning circuitry was not permanent, and the abnormality returned after weeks. This far-from-perfect direct current was soon supplanted by radio-frequency energy. With it, heat was produced locally and caused damage to the small area that was responsible for the abnormal heart rhythm. The change from uncontrolled tissue damage to a pinpoint-precision treatment was a true breakthrough. Soon several groups of physicians reported successful elimination of different types of SVT using this new technology in over 90 percent of cases. By removing the abnormal circuit, the heart-rhythm problem had been solved for good, and the patient was cured.[4]

Young people experiencing abnormal rhythms started getting evaluated and treated with ablation, removing the need for open-heart surgery. With their abnormal circuits eliminated, these patients required neither medicine nor follow up with the doctor to manage their condition. Cardiac ablation to treat SVT became one of the greatest successes in the history of cardiology.

Today, a patient can come in to their cardiologist, get an ablation, leave within twenty-four hours, and be back to work within forty-eight to seventy-two hours. During the procedure, the doctor puts a catheter in the heart, stimulates the heart to reproduce the abnormal rhythm, maps out the abnormal circuit, and destroys the abnormal circuit, all in one sitting. Every year several thousand patients undergo SVT ablation, which boasts a success rate upward of 95 percent.

Treating A-fib with ablation, however, is an entirely different story.

Knowledge Is Power

At this point in her years of dealing with A-fib, Mary knew the drill; her appointment was almost scripted, the same exchange year after year.

Dr. Susskind entered the room holding the chart in one hand, skimming over the details. Finally, he put down the chart but remained standing. "How many episodes of A-fib are you having these days?"

"The same amount as before: One every two months or so, lasting a few minutes. No changes.

"Are you taking your blood thinners?"

"Yes, religiously."

"Do you want me to get rid of your A-fib so you don't have to worry about it?"

"I'm not too worried about it; the episodes don't bother me much. As long as they aren't life-threatening, I'm okay carrying on with what I'm doing."

"The episodes aren't life-threatening," Dr. Susskind conceded, "but people with A-fib do have other issues, such as increased rate of heart failure, increased rate of dementia, and a shorter life span."

Mary smiled. She had asked the same question in response to this same warning, year after year: "Any mortality benefit for A-fib ablation in the new studies?"

Dr. Susskind smiled in return. "You set a high bar, don't you? No, there's no data on the possible mortality benefit of A-fib ablation in patients with an otherwise normal heart."

"Anything new in the field of A-fib ablation itself? Has the success rate increased to anywhere close to SVT ablation's?" she cheerfully pressed further.

"I wish. The success rate of SVT ablation is well over 90 percent, but A-fib ablation is about 70 percent." Dr. Susskind picked up her chart, getting ready to leave. "So, you want to continue as you are now and see me next year?"

"Yes," Mary told him. "If the episodes get really bothersome, I'll consider the ablation procedure, risks and all. So, I'll see you next year—sooner if things get worse. That okay with you?"

He nodded as he walked out the exam room door.

As Mary made her way back to the front of the office, she passed Corina making her way through the hallway, accompanied by the medical assistant. She smiled and offered a little wave in acknowledgment, but Corina stopped her with a hand on her arm. "Mary, I'm so sorry if this seems inappropriate, but I was wondering if you'd mind exchanging phone numbers so we connect. I'd love to continue the conversation we were having just now in the waiting room."

"Yes—I'd be happy to," she began, rummaging through her purse. "Here, let me give you my card," she said as she pulled one out, quickly scribbling her cell phone number on the back and handing it to Corina before waving a quick farewell and walking away.

The next day, Corina called Mary, and in short order they were meeting for coffee. After profusely thanking Mary for taking the time to meet up, Corina jumped right in to what was on her mind.

"Tell me if I've misunderstood you, Mary, but you said you've had A-fib for all these years but have *not* had an ablation?"

"Yes, that is correct," Mary smiled.

"Why not? Don't you want your A-fib cured?"

Mary nodded and then said, matter-of-factly, "Well, I've looked at the risks and benefits of the ablation procedure, read up a bit on it, and decided that it's not worth the risk for me, so I've decided to hold off."

"But what about the stroke risk?" asked Corina. "Patients with A-fib have a higher risk of stroke; doesn't that bother you?"

"Yes, I know patients with A-fib need to be on blood thinners to prevent stroke, but their need for blood thinners doesn't change after ablation. If I need blood thinners to prevent stroke before the ablation, I'll still need them afterward, even if the ablation is successful. It was never meant to prevent stroke. Ablation can't do that. Only blood thinners can."

Corina's face went pale. It was as if Mary had been reading straight from her medical chart. After a pause, Corina confessed, "I wish I'd known that before I went through my second ablation. I'd had one ablation that didn't work, followed by a second. *That* one seemed to have done the job, so I talked Dr. Susskind into getting me off the blood thinners. I was thrilled; I thought everything was headed in the right direction and my A-fib nightmares were behind me. Eight months after the ablation, I had a stroke."

"Oh dear!" Mary was truly shocked, given that it could have been prevented if Corina had continued the blood thinners.

"Yes," continued Corina gravely. "I went from being an active sixty-eight-year-old cycling enthusiast and world traveler to spending three months in a physical-rehab facility, struggling to regain my independence. Even now, there are still struggles." Not wanting to get sucked into this emotional quicksand, Corina quickly asked, "Are you not bothered by A-fib?"

"I do feel fluttering on and off, but only on rare occasions. It doesn't impact my life that much. If it did, if A-fib lessened my quality of life, ablation would become an option. But it doesn't. And if my quality of life is not being affected by A-fib, it seems like having such a risky, invasive procedure isn't worth it in the balance."

"But, Mary," said Corina, trying to take it all in, "I've heard people with A-fib don't live as long as people without A-fib. Wouldn't it be better to get the ablation done and resolve the A-fib, once and for all? This last visit, Dr. Susskind signed me up for my *third* ablation."

"Yes, it's true that people with A-fib don't live as long as those who don't have it, but the treatment with rate control does just as well as rhythm control. Given everything that could go wrong with rhythm control, I've decided to go with rate control."

"Rate control?" asked Corina, confused. "I don't know what that is. Can you explain?" Like any good CEO, she was comfortable seeking information from everyone to help her make sound decisions.

"*Rhythm* control is where you use procedures or medicines to keep your heart out of A-fib and in normal rhythm. *Rate* control's where you make sure your heart rate is well controlled but don't worry about reverting from A-fib to normal rhythm. Ablation is one kind of rhythm control, but taking medicine to keep your heart rate and pulse under control is called rate control."

"So, I'm on rhythm control, since they're trying to keep me in normal rhythm with ablations?"

"Yes, exactly," said Mary, nodding, "and I am on rate control because I'm not on any medicine to keep me *out* of A-fib but do take medicine to make sure my heart rate isn't high when I go *into* A-fib."

"And both options are equally good?"

"That's what the research shows. People who just control their heart rate whether they go into A-fib or not have the same longevity as anyone trying to keep out of A-fib. Ablation does not add years to your life compared to just controlling heart rate; there's zero mortality benefit. Every visit I ask Dr. Susskind if there's any more research to show ablation improves mortality, and every year the answer no, no, no—year after year. I tell him that if ablation could actually prolong my life I'd reconsider it, but rate control is just as good as rhythm control, so why take a chance?"

"Huh," said Corina, thoughtfully, "I see your point. They have to do monitors to detect my A-fib. I can't tell when I'm in it, so clearly it's not impacting my quality of life, and, like you said, the ablation isn't going to prolong my life span any more than controlling my heart rate with medicine will. I wonder if I should bother with the third ablation . . ."

"It's worth considering," offered Mary with a shrug. She didn't feel comfortable advising Corina against any procedure she was set on.

"I'm guessing you wouldn't do it if you were me?" Corina asked, grinning wryly.

A-fib Ablation

As early as the second century BC atrial fibrillation, called A-fib or AF, was recognized and mentioned in the historical literature, and then again in twelfth-century Spain by Jewish philosopher-physician Moses Maimonides. In the seventeenth century William Harvey observed and described it in animals. A-fib was identified as an irregular rapid beating in the upper chamber of the heart that could then cause the lower chamber to go fast in turn, thereby increasing heart rate and pulse. Patients suffering from A-fib reported a fluttering feeling, palpitations, and sometimes lightheadedness. However, as early as the eighteenth century, scientist Jean-Baptiste de Sénac had deduced that A-fib was not a disease by itself and had little to no long-term impact. The prevailing medical wisdom for the next two hundred years was that A-fib was a harmless abnormality and a nuisance, occasionally making patients uncomfortable but having no real effect beyond that.[5]

However, in 1978, data from the Framingham Heart Study—a long-term cardiac study of a group of people living in Framingham, Massachusetts, begun in 1948 and continuing today—made it clear that A-fib is associated with increased risk of stroke.[6] Within just a few years, through research on several thousand patients in numerous reports spanning continents, it became clear that use of blood thinners would mitigate risk of stroke. It also became clear that these patients would have to take blood thinners for the rest of their lives, regardless of whether they continued to have further episodes of A-fib or were in normal rhythm later.[7] After a patient experienced their first instance of A-fib, keeping the patient's heart in normal rhythm did not protect against stroke; only an ongoing use of blood thinners could achieve this. Once the stroke risk was mitigated, A-fib continued to be an irritant causing palpitations in a few, fatigue in others. In the large majority, however, it causes no symptoms.

In 1998, in Bordeaux, France, arrhythmia specialist and cardiac electrophysiologist Michel Haïssaguerre put catheters in human hearts to understand how A-fib starts. He noted that in patients with A-fib the initiating abnormal electrical activity originated from the pulmonary veins, which bring blood from lungs to the left upper chamber of the heart. To eliminate these triggers, he used the catheter-ablation technique now the norm in SVT ablations. Michel used this procedure with considerable success, and 62 percent of his patients thus treated remained free of A-fib without the need for medicine.[8] Soon it became clear that finding the initiating activity in A-fib was not important to treating the condition; rather, forming scar tissue around the pulmonary vein would electrically separate it and prevent the abnormal electrical activity from getting to the heart in the first place. The outcomes of this altered procedure were similar to Michel's initial successes, with 60 to 70 percent of patients undergoing the new procedure remaining free of A-fib one year after treatment. This was exciting news! Other electrophysiologists—arrhythmia specialists—started replicating and improving upon the technique.[9]

By the 2010s, the A-fib industry had reached five million patients strong and is still rising today.[10] Upon realizing its cash potential, industry specialists, hospitals, and physicians began exploiting A-fib accordingly. Variations in technical approach permitted by improved mapping technology, new catheters, and increased areas of targeted tissue destruction began to be attempted. And along with these improved technologies for ablation, newer gadgets for mapping and tools improving the procedure's safety were developed. New conferences began popping up targeting electrophysiologists looking to understand and fine-tune their technique.[11] As an attendee of one such gathering observed wryly, "You had to walk around with an umbrella not to be hit by a new tool or gadget marketed by the vendors at these conferences."[12] By 2011 the A-fib industry was estimated to be worth twenty-six billion dollars and was on track to rise by double digits every year.[13]

But observers began asking why patients were being subjected to a dangerous, invasive procedure that only enjoyed a success rate of only 60 to 70 percent when the disease itself is nothing more than a nuisance. Is it worth aggressively treating with ablation, they asked, when a patient can benefit as much by the use of medicine to maintain normal heart rate, regardless of the rhythm? This question was crucial and bothered some of the most experienced and astute doctors in the field.

The push by critical stakeholders for more aggressive treatments could only be justified if A-fib were proven to be more than a mere nuisance. One can only wonder if it's coincidental that around 1998 reluctance to resort to aggressive treatment was being assuaged by new data revealing that A-fib is a threat to the patient's longevity.[14] And over the years more reports on the dangers of A-fib were published, such that by 2002 the understanding was deeply entrenched that A-fib was a dangerous condition in and of itself.[15] Professional guidelines and consensus statements now began addressing the impact of A-fib on long-term mortality, and the industry, hospitals, industry-funded experts, and physician groups have since been sounding the alarm to the public about the dangers of A-fib.[16] This marketing surrounding A-fib created a partial justification for ablation.

We now had both a problem—A-fib, which was now considered dangerous—and a solution, albeit partial one—A-fib ablation. Professional societies continued to broadcast the dangers of A-fib and equally loudly broadcast the curative, ablation. More and more data on how to eliminate A-fib by ablation was being produced worldwide, and the quest to cure A-fib continued at a feverish pace.

Though *how* to eliminate A-fib had been researched extensively, *why* it was necessary to eliminate A-fib was still unclear. Despite A-fib's portrayal as a dangerous condition, it was unclear if eliminating A-fib and keeping patients in normal rhythm—that is, pursuing a *rhythm-control strategy*—mitigated this danger? Did rhythm-control strategy achieve anything more than accepting the existence of A-fib and controlling patient heart rate—or a *rate-control strategy*? Before A-fib ablation could be universally applied to every person with A-fib, two questions had to be answered: Is maintaining a normal heart rhythm better than controlling heart rate regardless of whether the heart is in A-fib or in normal rhythm? And does ablation reverse the impact of A-fib on longevity?

Numerous studies were undertaken to see whether A-fib needed to be eliminated by rhythm control or just managed at a lower heart rate with rate control.

The twenty-first century has seen more and more scientific evidence to suggest that, rather than eliminating A-fib, if one accepts A-fib and focuses on controlling heart rate with medications—a much easier, noninvasive, cheaper, and less-risky option—patients do equally well.

Here is a look at the conclusions from these numerous studies.

- In 2002, the AFFIRM investigation found that

  Management of atrial fibrillation with the rhythm-control strategy offers no improvement in survival over the rate-control strategy. In this study, restoring and maintaining sinus rhythm had no clear advantage over the strategy of controlling the ventricular rate and allowing atrial fibrillation to persist. . . .

  We did not find any benefit in association with the rhythm-control strategy. . . .

  None of the presumed benefits of rhythm control noted above were confirmed in this study. . . .

  The implication is that rate control should be considered a primary approach to therapy and that rhythm control, if used, may be abandoned early if it is not fully satisfactory.[17]

- In 2002, the RACE trial study found that

  Rate control is not inferior to rhythm control for the prevention of death and morbidity from cardiovascular causes. Rate control should therefore be considered much earlier in the course. . . .

  Effective preservation of sinus rhythm does not preclude the occurrence of cardiovascular events. . . .

  Among the patients treated with rhythm control, morbidity and mortality were similar whether sinus rhythm was maintained or atrial fibrillation recurred. . . .

  This finding suggests that the cardiovascular risk is not reduced with rhythm control even when sinus rhythm is maintained.[18]

- In 2009 the RECORDAF investigation found that

  The arrhythmia management strategy (rhythm control or rate control) was not predictive of clinical events (outcomes).[19]

- In 2011 a meta-analysis of four randomized controlled trials found that mortality and stroke were not significantly different in the two groups (rate control versus rhythm control), and hospitalizations were less frequent with rate control than with rhythm control.[20]

- And in 2016, the ORBIT-AF review found that

> Among patients with AF, rhythm control was not superior to rate control
> strategy for outcomes of stroke, heart failure, or mortality. . . .
>
> Randomized clinical trials on AF have shown no influence on survival,
> stroke or heart failure with rhythm control. . . .
>
> Physicians can educate their patients that there is no benefit in terms of
> incident stroke, heart failure, and death with a rhythm control strategy with
> antiarrhythmic drugs when compared to rate control for AF.[21]

However, every time one of these studies was published, the equally effective but non-revenue-generating rate-control strategy continued to be brushed aside. Well-documented complications of A-fib ablation were ignored.[22] And the rampant use of A-fib ablation continued.[23] Ablation enthusiasts proclaimed that in these studies, medicine was used to maintain normal rhythm but that these medicines are toxic. If ablation were to be used to restore and maintain normal rhythm, they argued, the rhythm-control strategy would prove to be better than the rate-control strategy. They claimed that the CABANA Trial—an ongoing study comparing ablation to medicine—would definitively prove once and for all that ablation is the great fix for A-fib. Meanwhile, the medical community continued to widely perform A-fib ablation, waiting on the study's results that they so hoped would justify the procedures they were already performing.

At the Heart Rhythm Society meeting in 2018, the CABANA Trial results were finally to be declared—the moment ablation enthusiasts had been waiting for. The meeting was held in the largest conference room the venue could provide, which had already filled to capacity fifteen minutes prior to the talk's scheduled start time. For the throngs of doctors who came afterward, it was standing room only. There was a definite air of enthusiasm; those in attendance had done ablations to help affected patients over the past two decades, and now they were eager to have all their efforts validated. They anticipated finally seeing the one slide in the results section that would show $p < 0.05$—or that ablation is a definitively better treatment for A-fib than drugs.

The stage was set, and the speaker walked in, beginning his talk with a cursory review of his many industry sponsors. He spent the next forty minutes discussing the dangers of A-fib—preaching to the choir. He then went on to present the methods of the study: About 1,100 patients used drugs to manage their A-fib, and the same number underwent ablation. Both groups were similar—like Mary and Corina. The assembled crowd could agree that the research had been conducted appropriately and that the results would be acceptable to everyone and applicable to all patients with A-fib. Once the results slide showed p < 0.05, they knew, there would be no doubters, and ablation would be known to be the undisputedly superior treatment for atrial fibrillation.

"And here are the results," the speaker announced, clicking to the one slide they were all there to see:

Death at five years in the two groups: $p = 0.3$, stroke at five years in the two groups: $p = 0.1$.[24]

No difference whether you do ablation or use medicine?
Let the spin begin . . .

APPENDIX

What Is the Normal Electrical System of the Heart?

As we have seen previously, the heart has its own electrical system. The heart's spark plug is the *sinoatrial node*. The *SA node*, as it's known, located in the right upper chamber, starts a normal heartbeat. From here, the electrical activity spreads to the two upper chambers. The electricity then conducts to the *atrioventricular junction*—or the *AV junction*—located between the upper and lower chambers. After a minor delay, the electricity spreads to the lower chamber, and the contraction of the lower chambers follows the electrical signal. In a normal heart, the upper chambers get the electrical signal and contract first. Moments later, the lower chamber receives the electrical impulses and contracts in a rhythmic, coordinated manner (see figure 8.3).

Our brain and body require fifty to one hundred beats of the heart per minute to be properly supplied with oxygenated blood, though a rare group of very athletic people requires fewer beats when they are resting.

What Are Arrhythmias?

Any pattern of electrical activity other than the normal pattern described above is considered abnormal and is called an *arrhythmia*. When the heart rate during the abnormal rhythm is faster than one hundred times per minute at rest—it is called *tachycardia*. *Supraventricular tachycardia*, or *SVT*, originates from the top chamber of the heart—the *atria*. *Ventricular tachycardia* originates from the bottom chambers of the heart—the *ventricles*.[25]

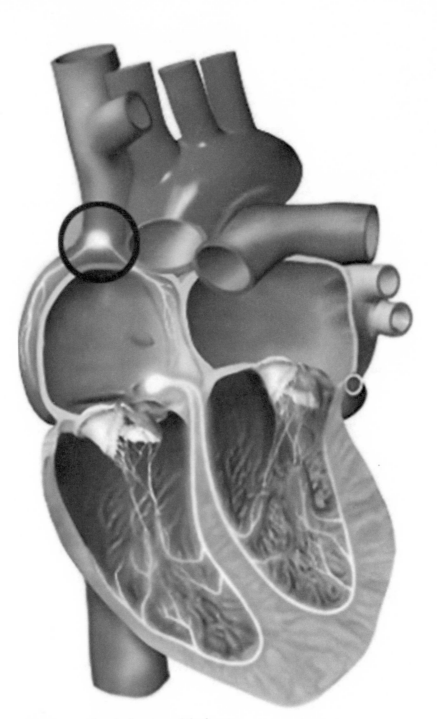

Figure 8.3.   Electrical system of the heart
Bruce Blaus

What Is SVT?

SVT is a type of abnormal heart rhythm where rapid heartbeats come from the top chamber of the heart.

What Are the Symptoms of SVT?

Typical symptoms of SVT include

- A feeling of fluttering in your chest that some people describe as palpitations
- A racing heartbeat (tachycardia)
- Chest pain
- Shortness of breath
- Lightheadedness or dizziness
- Sweating and
- Near-fainting or fainting.[26]

Is SVT Dangerous?

SVT is generally not a dangerous condition, though rapid fluttering of the heart may feel scary. Occasionally patients feel lightheaded, and, rarely, they pass out. SVT is not indicative of a heart attack, and having SVT does not put you at risk of a heart attack. SVT is not a life-threatening condition and has no negative impact on your survival.

What Causes SVT?

SVT is caused by the presence of an abnormal circuit in the heart. People are born with these abnormal circuits, but it may be years before they cause any problems. Depending on the location of the abnormal circuit, there are different types of SVTs.

What Are the Treatment Options for SVT?

Patients with SVT need treatment both when episodes happen and to prevent them from happening.

Immediate Treatment for an SVT episode

On occasion, an SVT episode may stop on its own. If it does not, try one of the following:

- Cough a few times.

If this does not work,

- Blow into a closed fist.

If this does not work,

- Take a deep breath, and hold it. Bear down hard with your stomach muscles as if you are having a bowel movement. Hold this strain for ten to fifteen seconds, then let go, and breathe normally again.

This last step may be repeated after a minute. If it does not work,

- Splash ice water on your face, or dip your face in ice-cold water.

If this still does not work, go to urgent care or an emergency room. They will make an assessment and likely give you an IV medicine to stop your SVT.[27]

Long-Term Prevention of SVT Episodes

SVT episodes can be prevented by medicine or with ablation. It may be appropriate to not take any steps to prevent SVT if the episodes are brief, they are infrequent (occurring less than once every six months), they stop on their own, or you are able to stop the episode with the above maneuvers. For frequent episodes that are long-lasting, cannot be stopped by the methods above, and require you to visit the emergency room very often, you may choose to take medicine daily or undergo an ablation procedure.

What Does an Ablation Procedure for SVT Involve?

You will be asked to not eat anything after midnight beforehand and to come to the hospital the day of the procedure. You will be prepared for the procedure in the prep area, after which you will be taken to the procedure room. Your doctor may choose to keep you comfortable with light sedation or may involve an anesthesiologist and let you fall asleep completely while they perform the procedure. Large IV lines will be placed in one or both of your femoral veins in your groin, and catheters will be passed through these IV lines into the heart. Your doctor will assess where the abnormal circuit causing your SVT is located. Once detected, the doctor will pass another catheter through to destroy the abnormal circuit. Repeat testing will be performed to make sure the SVT is no longer present, and the catheters will be removed. You will then be woken up and brought to the recovery area. The whole procedure lasts two to six hours, and you may be discharged to go home the same day or the day after.[28]

Are There Complications of SVT Ablation?

There are several potential complications of SVT ablation, depending on the location of the abnormal circuit, including

- Bleeding in the groin area at the site of the IV lines
- Damage to the blood vessels
- Accidental puncturing of the heart
- Accidental damage to the critical part of the electrical system of the heart (AV node) resulting in the need for pacemaker
- Clots in the legs
- Stroke and
- Rarely, death.[29]

Are There Different Types of SVT?

Yes, there are different types of SVT, depending on where in the upper chambers the abnormal circuit is located. You may be given a diagnosis of AVNRT, AVRT, AT, or atrial flutter.

What Is the Success Rate of SVT Ablation?

Depending on the location and type of SVT, the success of ablation ranges from 60 to 95 percent.[30]

Questions to Ask Your Doctor before SVT Ablation

- Based on my ECG, where is the abnormal circuit located?
- What is the expected success rate?
- What is the risk of pacemaker?
- What is the risk of stroke?
- Is medicine an alternative for me?
- Will I be awake or under general anesthesia?
- What symptoms will be resolved by ablation?

What Is Atrial Fibrillation?

Atrial fibrillation is a type of abnormal rhythm of the heart. In atrial fibrillation, instead of the heartbeat starting in the SA node, it starts in the left upper chamber in an erratic manner. It transmits to the AV junction between the upper and lower chamber and then to the lower chambers rapidly and irregularly, so your pulse feels rapid and irregular.[31]

What Are the Symptoms of A-fib?

Lots of patients do not feel any different when they are in A-fib (like Corina in the story above). However, some people are aware of their A-fib, and they experience

- Palpitation or fluttering of the heart
- Rapid heartbeat
- Shortness of breath with minimal exercise
- Lightheadedness or dizziness
- An unusual amount of fatigue
- Chest pain or pressure, a rare occurrence, and
- Also rarely, a feeling like they are going to pass out, or they do actually pass out.[32]

Can A-fib Cause a Stroke?

Patients with A-fib are at higher risk of stroke. A-fib along with other factors may increase the risk of stroke sufficiently to merit the use of powerful blood thinners. See table 8.1 to tally your risk factors and determine whether or not you require blood thinners.

If your total number of points in the CHA_2DS_2-VASc scoring system is 2 or greater, you may require powerful blood thinners to prevent a stroke.[33]

What Kind of Blood Thinners Should I Take to Prevent Stroke?

The following are the appropriate blood thinners to prevent stroke:

- Coumadin or warfarin
- Eliquis
- Pradaxa
- Xarelto
- Savaysa

Table 8.1. CHA$_2$DS$_2$-VASc Tool for Predicting Stroke Risk in Atrial Fibrillation

Condition	Point(s)
Congestive heart failure	1
Hypertension (even if controlled with medicine)	1
Age ≥ 75 years	2
Diabetes mellitus	1
Stroke or ministroke (TIA)	2
Vascular disease (coronary artery disease, previous heart attack, bypass surgery)	1
Age 65–74 years	1
Sex category (i.e., female sex)	1
	Total

Source: Adapted from Gregory Y. H. Lip, Robby Nieuwlaat, Ron Pisters, Deirdre A. Lane, and Harry J. G. M. Crijns, "Refining Clinical Risk Stratification for Predicting Stroke and Thromboembolism in Atrial Fibrillation Using a Novel Risk Factor-Based Approach: The Euro Heart Survey on Atrial Fibrillation," *Chest* 137, no. 2 (2010): 266.

Can I Use a Higher Dose of Aspirin to Prevent Strokes?

Aspirin does not prevent strokes associated with A-fib.

I Am on Aspirin and Plavix. Is That Sufficient to Prevent Strokes Associated with A-fib?

No. Studies have shown that aspirin and Plavix are not effective in preventing strokes associated with A-fib. Talk to your doctor about stopping either of these two medications when you start taking one of the blood thinners mentioned in the list above.

If I Am in Normal Rhythm, Do I Still Have to Take These Blood Thinners?

In patients with a history of AF, a normal rhythm does not prevent strokes; blood thinners do. Even if you are in normal rhythm, you will need to continue blood thinners if you are a candidate for them (i.e., if your CHA$_2$DS$_2$-VASc score is 2 or greater). Patients across various studies—and in this chapter's illustrative story—have had strokes even in normal rhythm if they quit their blood thinners.

What If I Bleed Easily?

In patients with a history of AF, blood thinners prevent strokes but may cause bleeding. Minor bleeds such as easy bruising are trivial compared to the risk of stroke. However, if you believe you have a tendency to have large bleeds, discuss the risks and benefits of using blood thinners with your doctor.

What Causes A-fib?

Possible causes of A-fib include

- Age (older people have an increased risk of A-fib)
- Hypertension or high blood pressure
- Heart disease (blockages in the heart artery, heart valve problems, weak heart muscles, etc.)
- Overactive thyroid
- Excessive use of stimulants such as caffeine, tobacco, or alcohol
- Lung diseases such as COPD or emphysema
- Infection
- Recent surgery
- Obesity and
- Other diseases such as sleep apnea, thyroid problems, kidney problems, etc.[34]

What Can I Do to Prevent A-fib?

To prevent A-fib,

- Maintain normal blood pressure
- Get checked and, if needed, treated for sleep apnea
- Use over-the-counter cold and cough medicine with caution
- Maintain a healthy weight
- Prevent excessive consumption of alcohol
- Avoid smoking and
- Increase your physical activity.

How Is A-fib Treated?

First and foremost, it is important to address the stroke risk and the need for blood thinners.

Next, it's important to determine your symptoms of A-fib and how bothersome they are. If you have no symptoms or very few symptoms from A-fib and it does not impact your quality of life, you may be a candidate for rate control.

If you have bothersome symptoms, you may be a candidate for either rhythm control or rate control. If your symptoms resolve or mostly resolve themselves with use of rate-control medicines and you do not have any side effects, you may choose a rate-control approach. If you continue to suffer through symptoms of A-fib despite rate control, rhythm control should be tried. This can be achieved with either medicine or ablation.[35]

What Kinds of Medicine Are Used for Rate Control?

- Beta-blockers such as metoprolol, carvedilol, propranolol, atenolol, bisoprolol, etc.
- Calcium channel blocker such as diltiazem, verapamil, etc., and
- Digoxin.

What Kinds of Medicine Are Used for Rhythm Control?

- Flecainide
- Propafenone (Rythmol)
- Sotalol (Betapace, Sorine)
- Amiodarone (Cordarone, Pacerone) and
- Dofetilide (Tikosyn).[36]

When Is It Appropriate to Consider A-fib Ablation?

If you are symptomatic and medicines for rate control or rhythm control have not worked, A-fib ablation is a good option. If you are symptomatic with A-fib and do not wish to use medicine for rhythm control, A-fib ablation is appropriate.

Ablation is *not* an alternative to the use of blood thinners to prevent a stroke. Maintaining sinus rhythm—or normal heart beat—does not reverse your risk of stroke.

How Successful Is A-fib Ablation?

Depending on the type of A-fib, about 50 to 70 percent of patients are free of A-fib one year after ablation. The number decreases as time goes on, meaning more patients start having A-fib again the longer it's been since they've had ablation. After multiple ablations, 80 percent of patients remain free of A-fib after five years.[37]

What Are the Risks of A-fib Ablation?

One out of fifteen patients undergoing A-fib ablation suffers from complications of the procedure. Death occurs in one out of two hundred to five hundred patients, stroke in one out of one hundred, and one out of forty has further heart problems as a complication of the procedure. Other problems may present in a small number of patients, including

- damage to the arteries
- damage to the veins and
- difficulty breathing.

Ablations among patients who are older than eighty years of age or have diabetes, a weak heart muscle, or lung problems have a higher complication rate than that mentioned above.[38]

What Does A-fib Ablation Involve?

You will be asked to not eat anything after midnight prior to the procedure and to come to the hospital on the day of the procedure. You will be prepared for the procedure in the prep area, after which you will be taken to the procedure room. You will most likely be under general anesthesia for the duration of the procedure. Large IV lines will be placed in both of your femoral veins in your groin area, and catheters will be passed through them into the heart. Your doctor will go from the right upper chamber of the heart to the left upper chamber by making a small hole. They will then use either a heat or cryo (cold) source to form scar tissue around all four pulmonary veins (veins that bring blood from the lungs to the heart). They may choose to burn or freeze some other areas as well, depending on your individual case. The catheters will be removed, and you will then be woken up and brought to the recovery area. The whole procedure lasts two to six hours, and you may be discharged the same day or the day after.

When Is a Pacemaker Used in Patients with A-fib?

If rate control is chosen and either the patient is unable to tolerate the medicine or the medicines used are not effective and the patient continues to remain at high rate, a pacemaker is appropriate. This is generally combined with a much shorter and safer ablation procedure, wherein the AV junction, the node connecting the upper and lower chamber of the heart, is destroyed. As a result, electrical activity in the upper chamber does not reach the lower chamber. The electrical activity in the lower chamber is generated through the pacemaker. Placing a pacemaker and then performing a short ablation of the AV junction does not eliminate the need for blood thinners for stroke prevention.

Some patients with A-fib also have slow heartbeats at times, and a pacemaker may be used in those situations also.[39]

What Questions Should I Ask My Doctor before Signing Up for A-fib Ablation?

- Which of my symptoms do you believe are related to A-fib?
- What benefit will I get from A-fib ablation?
- Is rate control an option for me?
- Is medical therapy for rhythm control an option for me?
- How many ablations do you do every year?
- What are the success rates in patients like me?
- Am I at a higher risk of failure of procedure than others?
- If I have recurrence of A-fib, what would be the next step?
- Do you have a surgeon on standby if the procedure goes awry?
- Will I be under anesthesia?

9

The Way Forward: The Home-Care Solution to Health Care

A clever person solves a problem. A wise person avoids it.

—Attributed to Albert Einstein

IT'S ALL CHAOTIC. WHAT IS ONE TO DO?

Which One Are You—Ron or Gary?

A shared childhood bridges many differences. The two men had grown up together in Macon, Georgia—a midsize town south of Atlanta—and had been friends for over fifty years. As with all friendships, life had pulled them apart at times and brought them together at others. Through it all, they continued to meet up for the annual weekend golf ritual they had started years ago. There had been six of them to start with, but life or death had come in the way for the other four. Nevertheless, Ron and Gary had continued with this tradition.

This year, Ron had bought them a package at the Sea Island golf resort in Georgia. He had said something about knowing someone and getting a deal, but Gary knew better; Ron had always been the giver of the group. Gary decided not to argue—and to make up for it when they met up.

He flew in from Oregon on Friday afternoon. Ron said he would swing through from Macon to pick him up at Savannah Airport so the two men could drive down to the resort together.

Gary found Ron waiting in his car outside arrivals. "Hey, hey! How's it going?"

"Great!" said Ron, in between bites of corn dog. "Hop on in." He knew they had to rush, or airport security would soon hassle them.

"How was the drive from home?" Gary asked, placing his duffel bag in the back seat.

"Good, very smooth." Ron started driving as soon as Gary was settled in. "There's no traffic in these parts at the best of times, but especially not when you know the back roads well." Ron had never left Macon, and the pair often joked he could probably drive around with his eyes shut.

"It's just as well you're driving; I have no idea!" said Gary with a laugh.

"Yeah, but you left for Oregon right after school. Things have changed around here over the years, that's for sure."

As they made the drive, an hour and change, they caught up on the previous year's events and the goings-on in each other's lives. This was a ritual too, like the audio version of a Christmas card.

Once they arrived at the resort, they checked in and decided to settle into their rooms and freshen up, planning to get together for dinner in two hours.

* * *

When Gary entered the dining area, Ron was seated at a table with a pint of beer in front of him. After they had greeted each other, Gary motioned to a waiter to request some water.

"Did you take a nap after that long plane ride? I bet you must be tired," Ron asked.

"Yeah, I am a little tired," acknowledged Gary. "We aren't so young anymore. But to keep my routine going, I decided to go for a quick jog for a few minutes and then freshened up."

Ron was impressed. "Boy, that's amazing! I'm tired just after the four-hour drive, I cannot imagine going out for a jog now, let alone after a long flight."

"I've been trying to get more exercise over the past two years, and . . ." Gary trailed off as he spotted the waiter hovering close by, waiting to take their orders.

"Good evening, gentlemen! My name is Chris, and I will be your server today. Can I tell you about our specials?" he asked, clearly following the script typical of a luxury resort.

"No, thanks—I know what I want," said Ron. He looked for confirmation to Gary, who nodded and offered a "Me, too."

"Excellent. What will it be, then, gentlemen?" asked Chris, deferentially.

"I'll have the steak, medium rare, with a baked potato on the side, please," said Ron with relish. "And could you please bring me another pint of beer?"

Gary wasn't surprised by his friend's order; Ron had always been the definition of a meat-and-potatoes guy.

"I'll have the sautéed vegetables," Gary said when Chris looked to him.

Ron gave his usual broad smile. "Is that going to be enough for you? I don't want you to be looking for food in the middle of the night!"

"I'll be fine," Gary assured him. "I had soup at the airport before you arrived."

"Guess you've picked up the habits of those Oregon people—exercising and eating healthy," Ron observed. "Good for you! But I'm a man of habits. You can't teach an old dog new tricks."

"Well, Mary and I are trying to pay attention to our health and do what we can." Gary's tone was cautious; he wanted to be mindful of his friend's feelings but also nudge him gently to improve his health. He looked forward to many more of these beloved trips together.

"My diabetes doctor has been pestering me, asking me to exercise and lose seventy-five pounds. Can you believe it? Seventy-five pounds! Truth be told, Barb and I joined the gym, but two weeks into it, life got in the way. Now I continue with my usual workout routine: I jump to conclusions, climb the walls, make mountains out of molehills, bend over backward, and run around in circles!" He let out the roaring laugh he had been known for since their high school days; Ron always found a way to make light of any situation.

"But seriously," he continued, "work gets so hectic these days I just don't have time to go to the gym." He didn't want Gary to get the impression he didn't care about his health at all, so he quickly added, "But I try to do everything else the doctor suggests for my diabetes. I'm taking my insulin regularly, and just to cover my bases, I'm also taking these chromium and cinnamon supplements. I read online that they're natural treatment options for diabetes."

Gary had looked into the natural-supplement industry in the past and knew how flimsy the science supporting it was.[1] However, he could tell Ron was getting a little defensive about his lifestyle choices and didn't want to put him on the spot. He quickly changed topics, and they continued to discuss their families throughout dinner.

Once they were through with their main course and the plates had been cleared, the waiter returned.

"Can I interest you gentlemen in desserts?"

"Yes!" said Ron decidedly, before Gary even had a chance to think about it. "I'll have your famous cheesecake." He turned to Gary with a wink. "I may have to take extra insulin, but I just can't resist their cheesecake."

"Of course," the waiter responded. Turning to Gary, he asked, "Shall I make that two?"

"Can I have a fruit dish instead?" Gary inquired.

"Yes, of course!" said the waiter, nodding. "Our seasonal fruits are very good this time of year; we're in peach country." With that, he took their orders to the kitchen.

While Gary had no desire to upset his friend, he was a little concerned about his food choices, especially given his diabetes.[2] But he had no intention of lecturing him on day one of their golf weekend and risking creating a disagreeable atmosphere for the rest of it. Gary changed the topic and inquired about some high school friends they had in common. The conversation carried them through the rest of the evening.

*   *   *

When Gary arrived the next morning, Ron was already waiting for him in a golf cart.

"Lovely day, isn't it?" Gary said, trying to hide his disappointment that they were not going to be walking such a beautiful course.

"Yes, I couldn't have ordered a better day myself," Ron replied. "This is going to be fun."

Over the next two days, the pair spent hours on the course chatting about life and reminiscing about the past. They discussed everything from weather and upcoming travels to world affairs, carefully steering clear of any thorny topics. By the end of the weekend, Ron was exhausted, and so were their conversation starters. They parted for home with plans to meet up the following year.

But next year, when it came time to plan their next reunion, Ron was unable to get away from work, though it disappointed him mightily. The friends arranged to reconvene the following year instead.

*   *   *

With all that had happened to Ron since the two men had last seen each other, Gary was just glad to be able to spend time with his friend the year after. They decided to meet in Macon, as Ron was worried about traveling too far and Gary wanted to catch up with other high school friends while there. It was decided they would golf at the Healy Point Country Club, which had recently undergone improvements under new management, according to Ron.

When Ron picked Gary up at the airport, he looked worn out, a shadow of his previous self. His skin was pale and sallow.

"You don't look a day older than when I saw you last!" Ron said, greeting Gary as brightly as ever.

"How have you been?" Gary asked, gently trying to divert attention from himself.

"Feeling okay! Recovery from the surgery has been an ordeal, that's for sure."

"Yes, but it was a big surgery; a three-vessel bypass is no joke. I bet your strong will and positive attitude is carrying you forward, though," Gary said, trying to keep Ron's spirits up. Though they moved on to talk about other topics, Gary quickly realized that Ron's health was going to be the eight hundred–pound gorilla in the room and resolved to explore it further over the weekend.

The next morning, Gary planned to meet up with Ron for breakfast, skipping his morning jog to do so. They got together at a local hangout where they had spent a lot of time during their high school days, and as always, Ron was already beaming from a nearby table when Gary arrived.

"Good morning!" Gary called to his friend. "You always impress me with your punctuality, it hasn't failed since school."

"Yeah, I guess you could say that. Did you sleep well?" Ron asked.

"Yes, I was a little tired from all the flight delays yesterday."

The waiter soon came and took their orders. This time, both of them ordered the same thing—coffee and oatmeal with strawberries and pecans.

"You are eating differently!" Gary blurted out.

"I wish I'd started sooner," Ron sighed.

Seeing an opportunity, Gary decided to not skirt around Ron's health issue any longer. "So, you were telling me over the phone how your heart disease was detected?"

"Oh, yes! It was the most fortunate thing. You'll remember we've always had very good doctors here. We're blessed!" As he told the story, Ron brightened up. "When I went for my annual physical, my doctor looked over everything and said that it all looked fine but ordered some tests to be sure.[3] And it turns out my diabetes results were not good."

"That's not good," Gary agreed, though he was not surprised.

"No," said Ron, "but it's funny how good things come out of bad situations. He said that my diabetes and weight were concerning, as at our age, heart disease is not uncommon. Thankfully, he mentioned this brand-new heart program they've started in the hospital and suggested that I get a thorough checkup and have them do a heart cath."[4]

"A heart cath? Isn't that where they put a tube in your heart and inject dye into it to take pictures?" Gary asked.

"I'm impressed! You know all about it, but I had no idea! I had to rely on the Internet. One fellow on a heart-health forum said they had performed the procedure and found a widow-maker of a blockage.[5] His post was so eye-opening that I just went along with what I was told. I met with the cardiologist, he explained what he was going to do, and they went ahead and checked out my coronaries. The doctor said my heart pumping was normal, but he found 70 percent blockages in three of my arteries."

"Oh, boy!" Gary exclaimed, shocked that such a condition could have gone unnoticed for so long.

"Yeah—good thing we looked, eh? I feel so fortunate that we have such great doctors in this town. Because of my diabetes, they said I couldn't have that many stents, so they recommended bypass surgery.[6] It was a real shocker!"

Their meals arrived. As Gary stirred his oatmeal, he grew thoughtful. "Hmm . . . some diet changes or medicine wouldn't have taken care of it?"

"No, a 70 percent blockage is serious business. The doctor didn't even want me to leave the hospital; he called the cardiac surgeon in town, and they operated the next morning!"

"That quick? It must have been serious!" Gary exclaimed, but privately he was doubtful. He had heard that unless you're seeking medical help for an ongoing heart attack, there is always time to get a second opinion on all heart surgeries. However, Ron had already gone through with it, so he stayed quiet. *Why bring up the past when it can't be changed?* he thought.

"Yep, they wasted no time, but within forty-eight hours they had to bring me back in to put in this pacemaker," he said pointing to a small lump on his left shoulder.

"You go walking in with nothing, and you come out a bionic man," Gary laughed. "How have things been since then? Are you feeling better? Do you have more energy?"

"I've been through physical rehab. It was a real struggle, but by the time they were done with me, I was walking two miles at a good speed."

"Have you continued with it?" Gary hoped that Ron had not returned to his old ways.

"Yes! You know, when I was in rehab, I was thinking about our last golf weekend and how active you were. I thought to myself, 'Gary would have had no trouble with this walking thing,' but then it occurred to me that you wouldn't have had heart issues to begin with, since you exercise so regularly."[7]

The waiter cleared the table, and Gary leaned forward, itching to continue the conversation.

"You would *think* so . . . that my jogging protects me from these sorts of heart troubles, I mean." Gary proceeded to tell Ron about his family history of heart disease and how they had found an increased cholesterol level at his last visit. The doctors had wanted to do a stress test.[8] "But as I explained to them," he continued, "I jog every day and have no trouble. Isn't that like a stress test? I told them I'd let them know if I had chest pain and that I didn't feel that any testing would help me right now."[9]

"And you've been okay?" Ron asked.

"Yes, fine. I also got a second opinion from another physician who doesn't work with any hospitals or anything. He advised me that if I am not having symptoms, there was no point doing any tests." Gary was proud that he had confirmed his hunch.

Ron was skeptical. "But isn't it better to just get it checked out?"

"I don't know. I was reading about it on the Mayo Clinic website—or maybe it was from Harvard. They said that if you don't have symptoms, the chances unnecessary procedures will uncover something lifesaving are way smaller than the chances they will lead you down the rabbit hole.[10] One test just leads to another and another . . ." Gary trailed off, realizing too late that he might be making Ron doubt his own condition.

"Hmm, maybe that's like mine . . . first a heart cath and then a bypass and then a pacemaker," said Ron, thoughtfully. "But maybe I genuinely needed them," he amended, wanting to feel justified in having followed the advice he'd received.

"Don't worry about it; you survived all of that, so it's time to look forward." Gary wanted to stop Ron's ruminating over it, though he regretted not having talked with him about it in the past.

"Yeah—time to look forward. My health is my number-one priority now!" Ron exclaimed.

"How do you plan to make it a priority?" Gary was not happy with mere lip service. He wanted to know if Ron had specific plans.

"I'll exercise daily and eat healthy," Ron declared.

Gary was trained in motivational interviewing and put this knowledge to use to ensure his friend was serious. He pointedly asked Ron about what exercise, where, how many times a week, and with whom, covering every little detail. He then proceeded to do the same thing with diet, and Ron quickly realized he might have to see a dietician.

"I believe in you, and I think you can do this!" said Gary, encouraging his friend. "This is a going to be a big change from the past."

"Yeah," agreed Ron, "I've discovered you're never too old to learn, especially not when your life depends on it!" The friends walked out of the café in high spirits.[11]

*   *   *

Over the weekend at the golf course, health was the major topic of conversation between the two men, though family and world affairs took their rightful place. Gary was pleased to note Ron tried to use the golf cart as little as possible between holes.

In the years that followed, the friends grew closer and talked frequently on the phone. Gary was impressed by the lifestyle changes that Ron had made and stuck with; he knew how difficult change could be but would often remind Ron that 90 percent of our health is down to what we do, and 10 percent is what doctors do.

Ron took this to heart, and five years later he was seventy pounds lighter, had gotten off his insulin, was walking four miles a day, and had not needed another stress test or heart cath. He continued to be active, though with age his run eventually slowed into a jog. He continued to eat healthily and visit with his friend once a year.

Many friends hope to grow old together, but Ron and Gary managed to do exactly that. BFFs indeed!

APPENDIX

Visiting a Doctor: How Do I Prepare for a Visit to the Cardiologist?

- Bring a friend or family member with you. Four ears are better than two, and it takes many repetitions for a message to be heard clearly. Doctors pack in a lot of information when they speak. Having someone else hear the information with you helps.
- Think about what you are suffering from. What symptoms are you having? When did they start? What triggers them? What relieves them? How does exercise affect them? Have they gotten better or worse over time? How long do they last? You should plan on describing them in detail.
- Bring any existing medication along with you. Make a list, and bring the medication bottles. This is the only guaranteed way to make sure the doctor knows what you are taking and what potential drug interactions to be concerned about with any new treatments.
- Write down your personal medical history, including all diseases you have been diagnosed with.
- Write down your surgical history.
- Write down any family history of heart disease, stroke, high blood pressure, diabetes, lung problems, or blood-related diseases. Has anyone in your family died unexpectedly at a young age?
- Think about how much you exercise. How often have you exercised in the past? Has there been a change in your exercise routine? If so, was it gradual or sudden?

- Write down if you or have you ever smoked? If so, how much? If you quit, when? Do you drink alcohol? If so, how much per week?

What Questions Should I Ask My Doctor When He Orders Tests or Recommends Procedures?

- What difference will the test make?
- What action will be taken if (a) the test is normal or (b) the test is abnormal? Note that if there is no difference in outcome, then there is no reason to undergo the test.
- If there is a procedure recommended, ask (a) How much will my life be prolonged by this procedure? (b) What quality of life improvement can I expect? and (c) If the only reason to perform a procedure is to prevent a future problem, how likely is the future problem to present, and how much risk am I being subjected to in order to prevent it?[12]
- If there is a procedure recommended, what are the possible complications? What percentage of patients have complications? Are there any factors that make me more or less likely to have these complications?
- Are there medications that can be used to treat the problem you are recommending a procedure for?
- If I start with medicine first and have side effects, can I then choose the recommended procedure later?
- Is doing nothing an option? What is the harm of doing nothing?

My Doctor Told Me about "Lifestyle Changes." What Exactly Are They?

Treatment for coronary artery disease usually involves lifestyle changes and, if necessary, drugs and certain medical procedures.

Your lifestyle largely determines how long you will live and the quality of life you will have. The impact that medical technology and procedures alone will have on your life is minor without changes to your lifestyle. Committing to a healthier life can be difficult; however, it is extremely rewarding.

There are certain key changes to your lifestyle that you can make that will have compounding healthy effects:

- Stop smoking: Smoking is a major risk factor for coronary artery disease, and there are many ways in which tobacco affects you negatively. If there is only one thing you promise to change, make the pledge to quit using all types of tobacco.
- Exercise: Being physically active has many advantages. It helps to control diabetes, improves your blood pressure and cholesterol levels, and helps

you maintain a healthy body weight. Starting is half the battle; once you keep with it, the energy to continue will miraculously appear. Remember, energy begets energy! Over time, you will find it easier to increase the distance and time of your walking, jogging, and running.

- Maintaining an ideal body weight: Obesity increases the risk of heart disease. Weight loss can be a struggle for some, but it will be lifesaving for many.
- Controlling your diabetes: Diabetes is almost synonymous with heart disease. If you control your diabetes, you will also control your chances of coronary artery disease.
- Keeping your blood pressure under control: Your target blood pressure should be less than 130 mm Hg (millimeters of mercury) for the upper number and 90 mm Hg for the lower number. Under certain circumstances, your doctor may specify a lower target blood pressure. If your blood pressure is consistently high, initial lifestyle changes and later medication may be needed to achieve your target blood pressure.
- Improving your cholesterol values: Depending on your risk factors, you may need to get a routine cholesterol check. Most people should aim for an LDL cholesterol (bad cholesterol) level below 130 mg/dL (milligrams per deciliter).[13]
- Eating healthy foods: A plant-based, heart-healthy diet rich in fruits, vegetables, whole grains, legumes, and nuts has been shown to decrease the likelihood and impact of heart disease. Avoid saturated fat, trans fats, excess salt, excess sugar, and excess alcohol.
- Managing stress: Reduce your stress as much as possible. Practice healthy techniques for managing stress, such as muscle relaxation and deep breathing. In addition, it may benefit you to look into a mindfulness-based stress-reduction program and get training in mindfulness techniques.
- Adopting optimism: Optimists have a quarter of the heart-disease rate of pessimists. Find ways to develop your optimism. If you can see the glass as half full, it will only get fuller!

How Much Do Lifestyle Changes Impact Heart Disease?

In a recent report, thirty-two regions of the United States were assessed for smoking, diet, and physical inactivity. The numbers of stress tests, heart caths, and angioplasties or bypass surgeries performed in these regions were also compared. Finally, overall death rate and rates of death related to heart disease were compared. A strong connection was found between poor behaviors involving diet, exercise, and smoking and death due to heart disease. Angioplasty and bypass surgeries did not explain the difference in overall death rates or heart disease–related deaths.[14]

In other words, it isn't what your doctor does that impacts how long you will live but, rather, your smoking, diet, and exercise habits. It has been proven in several studies that life expectancy does not depend on the health-care system but on the life you lead at home. If smoking, diabetes, high blood pressure, and obesity were eliminated, heart-disease death rates could be cut in half. There is no pill, procedure, or surgery that could have that kind of impact. Therefore, if you want to live a longer and healthier life, make these lifestyle changes. Doctors and health-care systems have little to do with how long you will live, except in emergencies.

How About Preventive Cardiac Testing? Isn't It Better to Catch a "Widow-Maker" Early?

A number of research studies have shown that preventive stress tests lead to more tests and more procedures without any impact on longevity. In places where more stress tests are available, people naturally get more stress tests, and, by extension, more heart caths and more stents, even when patients have low risk factors. There is no improvement in longevity in these places compared to those places where fewer stress tests are performed. A "widow-maker" is rarely actually stumbled upon, whereas unnecessary testing frequently leads to more unnecessary testing and procedures. It is far more likely that this procedure to search out any possible widow-makers will result in life-changing complications than it is likely that you will find this rare disease that has gone undetected.[15]

My Physician Wants to Perform a Stress Test, but I Have No Symptoms. What Should I Do?

There is no data to show that stress tests or other more-invasive procedures improve longevity in the long run, but they do generally increase the chances of requiring yet another test and then another procedure. According to professional societies, there is no role for stress tests in asymptomatic patients.[16]

How about Stress Testing before a Surgery?

Other than in surgery on the major blood vessels of the chest and abdomen, there is no data to show that anyone needs stress testing prior to surgery. If your physician refuses to clear you for surgery without getting these tests, get a second opinion.[17] If you have symptoms of chest pain or shortness of breath, you may be better off getting that checked out regardless of whether or not you need surgery.

How about the Use of Supplements? What Role Do These Play in Managing My Health?

Herbal remedies and natural supplements are heavily marketed, and many testimonials are often provided as proof of the positive impact these supplements have. However, a large majority of these supplements have few valid research studies to prove their efficacy. Furthermore, since they are not tested or monitored by the FDA as closely as other medications, the safety of taking them remains questionable.

Some of these herbal supplements may have a dangerous impact on heart problems. Serious interactions with other heart-related medications have been reported with these supplements. You should not use supplements without first checking with your doctor.

The National Center for Complementary and Integrative Health is an excellent resource for summaries of medical studies and their conclusions regarding numerous herbal and natural supplements. Since the agency's only goal is to help consumers make better choices, they provide unbiased information, whereas websites touting the positive impact of natural supplements that also sell them have an inherent bias toward any positive impact their product may provide. These websites ignore all the negatives and safety concerns surrounding these supplements, so it is not wise to rely on vendors for information on the impact of supplements or any other medication. Vendor websites can be easily identified: They usually include a button for the "Cart" and a request for your credit card number.

What Medications Are Used for Heart Disease?

If you have blockages in the heart arteries, the following medications can be used to treat them:

- Aspirin
- Beta-blockers such as metoprolol
- Nitroglycerin, either as needed or daily
- Cholesterol-lowering medicine
- ACE inhibitors (or angiotensin-converting-enzyme inhibitor) such as lisinopril and
- ARBs (or angiotensin-receptor blocker) such as losartan.

Epilogue

Heart-to-Heart

Until he extends his circle of compassion to include all living things, man will not himself find peace.

—Albert Schweitzer[1]

Contemporary medicine today is marred by many issues. The stories you have read in this book speak of the wonders of medical science going awry because of reckless, indiscriminate, and hasty use of tests and treatments. There are many contributors to this problem, with few winners and numerous losers.

HOW CAN SUCH SMART DOCTORS
MAKE MISTAKES LIKE THIS?

In a typical visit, doctors use their medical knowledge and past experience to make a diagnosis and then decision regarding the treatment plan. Their expertise allows them to develop mental shortcuts or rules of thumb to help process a lot of information in a quick and efficient manner. For example, if fever and cough has persisted for a week, look for pneumonia; in weight loss and cough lasting over three months in a smoker, look for lung cancer. These rules of thumb help decision-making and, in the majority of the circumstances, serve doctors well. However, these very rules of thumb may introduce errors in judgment due to their potential to narrow the focus on two or three aspects of the patient's history while ignoring others. These fallacies made by overrelying on established rules of thumb are called *cognitive biases.*[2]

For many of us, a visit to the doctor always seems rushed. Patients feel that they have to squeeze as much as possible into a fifteen-minute time slot. In such a rush, as soon as the patient utters the first or second symptom, the doctor seizes on a treatment path charted out in that direction. Here the *order effect,* a type of cognitive bias, creeps in. The order in which information is received impacts the way the doctor processes it to reach the diagnosis.[3]

In chapter 2, when Carl's fatigue drove him to the doctor's office and when questioned he happened to mention some muscle soreness, Sean, the physician's assistant, zeroed in on "chest pain," and the course for Carl's treatment was set—erroneously, as it turned out in the end. In shorter office visits, doctors frequently make hasty preliminary diagnoses based on the order in which information is provided. They then recommend tests to confirm this diagnosis.

Any test result that even partly confirms the doctor's initial impression will only further convince the doctor that the original diagnosis was correct. This is where the doctor becomes a victim of *confirmation bias,*[4] the cognitive error whereby any information that serves to validate the initial impression is highlighted while other possibilities are discredited. In chapter 3, Jack, the cardiologist, had decided that blockages in the heart arteries were causing his friend Saul's fatigue. The borderline blockage was enough to confirm Jack's belief, and other probable causes of fatigue were immediately taken off the table. Again, erroneously.

Once there are pieces of information that match one diagnosis, thinking stops. This is the cognitive bias of *premature closure.*[5] In chapter 6 we saw that when Patricia's fatigue was being assessed by her medical team, once her low heart rate was noted, no other factors were considered. Patricia's other symptoms, her previous heart rate, and the tests performed in the past by her long-time primary-care physician, Dr. Saleh, were all overlooked, and a snap judgment of low heart rate causing the fatigue was made. With a detailed conversation, an open mind, and an ongoing assessment, the doctors could have recognized that her low heart rate had no connection to her fatigue, and her unnecessary pacemaker implantation could have been avoided. Premature closure led to the unnecessary pacemaker placement.

In our society of go-getters, action is revered. Among doctors, who tend to have a type A personality, the inclination to act is even more pronounced. Once they see the possibility acting on or treating a condition, other options are ignored.

Patients who also share in this inclination for action feel better when they see that "something is being done." The more visible the effort, the more comforted the patient. However, not all action is scientifically justified or needed.

Remember that urge to take a longer route to avoid sitting in a traffic jam? That's *action bias*,[6] which is a cognitive error in truth because inaction would have been a more rational choice to reach your destination faster. Action bias is commonly observed in medicine. When the data are unclear, it takes a lot of wisdom and patience to hold back on acting and treating, even if there is a good chance time will heal what ails the patient.

In chapter 7 when Jessica experienced postpartum heart problems, Dr. Shankman wanted to act to protect her life. Though half the patients in Jessica's situation get better within a few months and it is unlikely that waiting would do them any harm, the urge to act was so strong that her doctor rushed Jessica to get an ICD in a hurry. Jessica became a victim of action bias and suffered from a hastily placed ICD and its complications.

Numbers are dry; stories are powerful. The chance of dying from a shark attack is one in 3,748,067—less than the chance of dying by falling vending machine, dog attack, lightning, or car crash. However, if you avoid getting into the water on your beach vacation after reading or hearing about shark attacks on the news, you understand the power of stories. Though we would hope our doctors would be guided by scientific studies and professional-society guidelines when diagnosing and treating us, doctors, like the rest of humanity, are swayed by stories. They remember and are consciously or subconsciously guided by patient stories, especially where there was a bad outcome. This is known as *availability bias*.[7] The story of a patient who suffers a bad outcome is at the forefront of the doctor's mind and so is easily available for recall, which ends up dictating the course of action in future cases.

In chapter 1, one of Dr. Shandra's healthy patients had suffered a complication during knee surgery. The impact of that event loomed so large in the doctor's mind that he wanted to avoid that fate at all costs. As a result, he was ordering stress tests on all of his patients to uncover any silent heart problems, despite society guidelines, and clear evidence showing the negative impact of the indiscriminate use of stress tests. As a result, his patient Barbara suffered because of a stress test she did not need.

If you believe in UFOs, a photograph of an unusual shape in the sky or an unexpected flash of light provides strong "evidence" that UFOs are real. The same photograph appears unremarkable to the nonbeliever and may even further convince them that UFOs do not exist. This is known as *belief bias*,[8] and doctors are not immune from it. While more and more scientific evidence shows that stents are not as helpful outside of an emergent heart attack situation, interventional cardiologists like Saul's' doctor, Jack, are incredulous. Despite ample evidence to the contrary, they continue to persevere in their belief that having an unblocked open artery is the only way to a long and healthy life. They refuse to believe the clear scientific evidence showing that patients receiving medicines do just as well as those receiving a stent. These doctors' inability to appropriately regard the data leads to the indiscriminate use of stents due to both explicit and implicit belief in their lifesaving capacity.

When doctors rush through patient visits, they also rush their thinking process. This invites cognitive errors that contribute to poor decision-making and treatment plans that may or may not be appropriate for the patient.

> It is difficult to get a man to understand something, when his salary depends on his not understanding it.
>
> —Upton Sinclair[9]

In addition to these cognitive biases, economic considerations also affect decision-making. The health-care system is set to reward actions, tests, and procedures disproportionately compared to the remuneration health-care providers receive for a clinic visit. Action pays more than observation, and surgeries profit more than conversations. So even when the action taken may not have an impact on either the quality or quantity of patient life, there is an economic drive to perform more tests or procedures. Doctors who perform more tests and procedures both make more money and generate more money for their hospitals.[10] They are cherished as leaders and applauded as rainmakers and are often considered gifted and talented. Patients believe that more tests and treatment will lead to better outcomes,[11] so doctors who perform extra testing—whether that testing is scientifically justified or not—are put on a pedestal by patients and hospitals alike.

Doctors who provide scientifically justified care observe when appropriate and act when justified. However, they also leave action-primed patients confused, hospital administrators frustrated, and their own paychecks smaller.

THE PATIENT EXPERIENCE

When patients interact with doctors, the patient expects a humane interaction with an expert. They look for someone who can understand their situation, empathize with their experience, share in their concerns, and care about them and their families.[12] Instead, interaction with the health-care system has become a scary prospect. A frustrating call to the doctor's office, being put on hold, being offered a clinic appointment four to six weeks later, and dealing with the insurance company all take their toll on a patient—and all this before they even reach the doctor's office! Once there, filling out the paperwork, hoping to see the doctor in a timely manner, and the anxiety of understanding medical jargon make for an agitating experience. By the time the patient is finally in front of the doctor, they're already frustrated and confused.[13] All the questions they had intended to ask to the doctor are scattered from their mind like leaves in the wind, and they have to collect themselves, remember everything relevant, and ask all the pertinent questions that have been bothering them in a short period of time.

In a fifteen-minute appointment, when the doctor comes in, there is a sense of urgency in the room. The doctor has to get to the next patient and often stands to talk, with no time to sit and converse. Their eyes shift from the computer to the patient, and their barrage of questions, rapid-fire diagnoses, and treatment recommendations—that could be in a foreign language for all their comprehensibility—all in such a sterile, clinical environment, leaves the patient yearning for more. The connection with the doctor is insipid; the system and process appear soulless and heartless.[14]

THE PHYSICIAN EXPERIENCE

When entering medical school, students are expected to submit a personal statement explaining why they want to be doctors. When applying for an internship, they are asked to explain why they opted for a particular placement. This same line of questioning continues throughout their training. Ninety-nine percent of future doctors talk about the desire to take care of people, serve humanity, feel a connection with patients, and relieve their patients' pain and suffering. And then . . . they graduate.

They become part of a practice and jump into the business of medicine. Soon they have to worry about overheads, payroll, rent, and utilities. Urged to increase their productivity, they put multiple patients into the same time slot, and soon the fifteen-minute patient visit becomes the new norm. In this abbreviated slice of time, they are expected to get the patient's "detailed" medical history, examine them, try to determine a diagnosis, recommend tests or treatments, explain the benefits of the treatment plan, and complete their notes, with all the pertinent details added in. Between patients, doctors respond to queries over the phone, check lab results that have come in, go through notes that other doctors have sent them, and coordinate patient care. Some doctors have additional duties at the hospital and have to go back-and-forth between seeing patients in the clinic and in the hospital. Then there is the on-call schedule, requiring them to spend sleepless nights working and then going back on duty the next day. Doctors are stretched thin, expected to be at two places at the same time, with ever-increasing metrics and parameters of patient satisfaction to meet. Each encounter with a patient is assessed and rated on every aspect of the interaction. If they do not meet the required scores, the administrators are quickly knocking on their door for a "conversation."[15]

In this three-ring circus, the doctor's original, best intentions to understand their patient's concerns is lost, and any hope of meaningful connection they yearn to have with their patient vanishes. The desire to care and to cure has disappeared. For many conditions, the limits of science make a cure a distant hope, and the health-care system makes care little more than an advertisement billboard. All of this fatigues, stresses, and angers doctors.

Burdened by their hectic schedules and the system's misplaced priorities, doctors suffer in mind, body, and spirit and eventually cave to the pressure and become task-oriented. The unsolved mysteries of patient health, the feeling of helplessness bred by bad outcomes despite a doctor's best efforts, and the inevitable deaths all lead to cynicism. Doctors start losing faith in their ability to make any real change to a patient's outcome, and this existential crisis only adds to their physical fatigue and mental agony. When doctors are stressed and frustrated, compassion and caring become the first victims.

Soon, the doctor is no longer available to their patients. Commitment dwindles; depression increases, authenticity abates; anxiety spikes.[16] The doctor becomes emotionally distant, withdrawn and detached, treating diseases, not patients. It takes one human to see another, but under stress, fatigue, and near-burnout, the doctor leaves the kind human being behind, bringing only the technical expert to work while the mind and spirit stay back. Tasks and processes take over; care and compassion lag behind. The heart that can touch another heart is missing.

This disconnect is soon noted by the patients, both consciously and subconsciously. They become reluctant to return to the clinic, are unlikely to follow instructions, and likely grow dissatisfied with the care they receive. This negative energy in turn impacts the doctor, who notices the rut and feels the burnout, and the rate of errors and the possibility of lawsuits increase. The doctor considers leaving the job—or worse, seeking solace in alcohol or drugs, starting a death spiral for the caring and compassionate connection between the doctor and the patient that had once inspired them to enter the field in the first place.[17]

WHERE IS THE BRIDGE TO CONNECT THE TWO?

The Dalai Lama, a simple man with a deep understanding of human suffering, once said that "Real care of the sick does not begin with costly procedures; it begins with the simple gifts of love, affection, and concern."[18] Patients seek another human being with expertise who understands their suffering and is committed to trying to relieve it. They yearn for care first and a cure if possible. In fragile times of anxiety and stress, they crave a human touch to their care more than ever. As the adage goes, they don't care how much you know until they know how much you care.

When they encounter doctors who introduce themselves and shake their hand, patients feel like equals and sense they are respected. When a doctor sits down and makes eye contact, they see that the doctor is engaged and feel better able to provide a more complete history. When a doctor speaks from the heart, patients feel important, cared for, and understood. When they know that the doctor is emotionally open and available, they reveal their own hearts, inner fears, and concerns. A doctor who is truly present is able to calm and comfort the patient and their family. In these moments, a doctor sees a person and not cluster of diseases. They understand the human behind the gown, and the potential for their own cognitive errors in diagnosis and treatment decrease. Now there is an opportunity for two-way communication with joint problem-solving and decision-making. With this openness, judgment improves and diagnoses are more accurate. Tests and procedures are ordered more judiciously. When there is more heart, more care, and more empathy, patient satisfaction and self-care increases, pain levels decrease, and recovery speeds up.[19]

Patient satisfaction and physician satisfaction are intricately intertwined. When the focus shifts from the disease to the person coping with disease, the impact is mutually rewarding. When the doctor sits down and talks as one human to another, providing hope and courage, they sense the privilege of being there for another human. In such moments, they can observe the gratitude in the eyes of the patient, and when they stay rather than withdrawing, the humility of serving a fellow human takes center stage. When they offer support rather than detachment, the sense of meaning in work comes back.[20] When patient satisfaction improves, so does physician satisfaction. At this stage, the positive impact on reputation, public perception, and paycheck becomes a mere sidenote.

Heart-to-heart conversation between patient and doctor helps build a relationship, and it is within this relationship that patients find healing and physicians find meaning.

> And now here is my secret, a very simple secret: It is only with the heart that one can see rightly; what is essential is invisible to the eye.
>
> —Antoine de Saint-Exupéry[21]

Notes

INTRODUCTION: WHY DO I NEED THIS BOOK?

1. Attributed to Thomas Edison.

2. Salim Yusuf et al., "Effect of Coronary Artery Bypass Graft Surgery on Survival: Overview of 10-Year Results from Randomised Trials by the Coronary Artery Bypass Graft Surgery Trialists Collaboration," *The Lancet* 344, no. 8922 (1994): 563–70.

3. American Heart Association, "Lifestyle Changes for Heart Attack Prevention," Heart.org, last reviewed July 31, 2015, http://www.heart.org/HEARTORG/Conditions/HeartAttack/LifeAfteraHeartAttack/Lifestyle-Changes-for-Heart-Attack-Prevention_UCM_303934_Article.jsp.

4. Dartmouth Atlas Project, "General FAQ," visited January 23, 2018, https://www.dartmouthatlas.org/faq/.

5. Elliott S. Fisher et al., "The Implications of Regional Variations in Medicare Spending. Part 1: The Content, Quality, and Accessibility of Care," *Annals of Internal Medicine* 138, no. 4 (2003): 273–87, http://annals.org/aim/fullarticle/716066/implications-regional-variations-medicare-spending-part-1-content-quality-accessibility.

6. Sarah L. Goff et al., "How Cardiologists Present the Benefits of Percutaneous Coronary Interventions to Patients with Stable Angina: A Qualitative Analysis," *JAMA Internal Medicine* 174, no. 10 (2014): 1614–21, https://jamanetwork.com/journals/jamainternalmedicine/fullarticle/1898875.

7. Elisabeth Rosenthal, *An American Sickness: How Healthcare Became Big Business and How You Can Take It Back* (New York: Penguin Press, 2017), passim.

8. Ezekiel J. Emanuel, "Are Good Doctors Bad for Your Health?" *New York Times*, November 21, 2015, https://www.nytimes.com/2015/11/22/opinion/sunday/are-good-doctors-bad-for-your-health.html.

9. M. J. Barger-Lux and R. P. Heaney, "For Better and Worse: The Technological Imperative in Health Care," *Social Science and Medicine* 22, no. 12 (1986): 1313–20.

10. Andrew Y. Chang et al., "Evaluating the Cost-Effectiveness of Catheter Ablation of Atrial Fibrillation," *Arrhythmia and Electrophysiology Review* 3, no. 3 (2014): 177–83, https://www.ncbi.nlm.nih.gov/pmc/articles/PMC4711535/.

11. Thomas Jefferson to Caspar Wistar, June 21, 1807, in *The Works of Thomas Jefferson in Twelve Volumes,* Federal edition, collected and ed. Paul Leicester Ford (New York, London: G. P. Putnam's Sons, 1904–1905).

12. Attributed to Benjamin Franklin.

CHAPTER 1: STRESS TEST: IS WHAT'S GOOD FOR THE GOOSE GOOD FOR THE GANDER?

1. Sarah McBride, "The Real Me," *The Huffington Post,* May 9, 2012, https://www.huffingtonpost.com/sarah-mcbride/the-real-me_b_1504207.html.

2. Harold E. B. Pardee, "An Electrocardiographic Sign of Coronary Artery Obstruction," *Archives of Internal Medicine* 26, no. 2 (1920): 244–57; Guy Bousfield, "Angina Pectoris: Changes in Electrocardiogram during Paroxysm," *The Lancet* 192, no. 4962 (1918): 457–58; Bernard S. Oppenheimer and Marcus A. Rothschild, "Electrocardiographic Changes Associated with Myocardial Involvement with Special Reference to Prognosis," *JAMA* 69, no. 6 (1917): 429–31.

3. W. Bruce Fye, "A History of the Origin, Evolution, and Impact of Electrocardiography," *American Journal of Cardiology* 73, no. 13 (1994): 937–49.

4. *Wikipedia,* s.v. "Robert A. Bruce," last modified January 17, 2018, https://en.wikipedia.org/w/index.php?title=Robert_A._Bruce&oldid=820858904; Myrna Oliver, "Robert Bruce, 87; Researcher Developed Treadmill Stress Test," *LA Times,* February 16, 2004, http://articles.latimes.com/2004/feb/16/local/me-bruce16.

5. Arthur M. Master, Rudolph Friedman, and Simon Dack, "The Electrocardiogram after Standard Exercise as a Functional Test of the Heart," *American Heart Journal* 24, no. 6 (1942): 777–93.

6. *Wikipedia,* s.v. "Treadmill: Treadmills for Punishment," last updated January 10, 2019, https://en.wikipedia.org/wiki/Treadmill#Treadmills_for_punishment.

7. R. A. Bruce et al., "Exercise Testing in Adult Normal Subjects and Cardiac Patients," *Pediatrics* 32, no. 4 (1963): 742–56.

8. Harvard Men's Health Watch, "Cardiac Exercise Stress Testing: What It Can and Cannot Tell You," Harvard Health Publishing, updated August 22, 2018, https://www.health.harvard.edu/heart-disease-overview/cardiac-exercise-stress-testing-what-it-can-and-cannot-tell-you.

9. Ibid.

10. Kristin M. Sheffield et al., "Overuse of Preoperative Cardiac Stress Testing in Medicare Patients Undergoing Elective Noncardiac Surgery," *Annals of Surgery* 257, no.1 (2013): 73–80, https://www.ncbi.nlm.nih.gov/pmc/articles/PMC3521863/pdf/nihms409211.pdf.

11. S. Andrew Sems, Erik C. Summers, and Traci L. Jurrens, "Cardiac Stress Testing Has Limited Value Prior to Hip Fracture Surgery" (paper #49, presented at the 23rd Annual Meeting of the Orthopaedic Trauma Association, Boston, October 18–20, 2007).

12. Joseph A. Ladapo, Saul Blecker, and Pamela Sylvia Douglas, "Physician Decision Making and Trends in the Use of Cardiac Stress Testing in the United States: An Analysis of Repeated Cross-Sectional Data," *Annals of Internal Medicine* 161, no. 7 (2014): 482–90.

13. Ibid.

14. Daniel W. Mudrick et al., "Downstream Procedures and Outcomes after Stress Testing for Suspected Coronary Artery Disease in the United States," *American Heart Journal* 163, no 3. (2012): 454–61, https://www.ncbi.nlm.nih.gov/pmc/articles/PMC3886123/.

15. Serge C. Harb et al., "Exercise Testing in Asymptomatic Patients after Revascularization: Are Outcomes Altered?" *Archives of Internal Medicine* 172, no. 11 (2012): 854–61, https://jamanetwork.com/journals/jamainternalmedicine/fullarticle/1151706.

16. Daniel W. Mudrick et al., "Patterns of Stress Testing and Diagnostic Catheterization after Coronary Stenting in 250 350 Medicare Beneficiaries," *Circulation and Cardiovascular Imaging* 6, no. 1 (2013): 11–19, https://www.ahajournals.org/doi/full/10.1161/CIRCIMAGING.112.974121.

17. Nael Aldweib et al., "Impact of Repeat Myocardial Revascularization on Outcome in Patients with Silent Ischemia after Previous Revascularization," *Journal of the American College of Cardiology* 61, no. 15 (2013): 1616–23, http://www.onlinejacc.org/content/61/15/1616; Bimal Ramesh Shah et al., "Patterns of Cardiac Stress Testing after Revascularization in Community Practice," *Journal of the American College of Cardiology* 56, no. 16 (2010): 1328–34, http://www.onlinejacc.org/content/56/16/1328; Bimal Ramesh Shah et al., "Use of Stress Testing and Diagnostic Catheterization after Coronary Stenting: Association of Site-Level Patterns with Patient Characteristics and Outcomes in 247,052 Medicare Beneficiaries," *Journal of the American College of Cardiology* 62, no. 5 (2013): 439–46, http://www.onlinejacc.org/content/62/5/439; Vinay Kini et al., "Clinical Outcomes after Cardiac Stress Testing among US Patients Younger than 65 Years," *Journal of the American Heart Association* 7, no. 6 (2018): e007854, https://www.ahajournals.org/doi/10.1161/JAHA.117.007854.

18. Xiaoyan Huang and Meredith B. Rosenthal, "Overuse of Cardiovascular Services: Evidence, Causes, and Opportunities for Reform," *Circulation* 132, no. 3 (2015): 205–14, https://www.ahajournals.org/doi/full/10.1161/CIRCULATIONAHA.114.012668; Sarah Jane Reed and Steve Pearson, "Choosing Wisely® Recommendation Analysis: Prioritizing Opportunities for Reducing Inappropriate Care," Institute for Clinical and Economic Review, [May 2015], http://www.choosingwisely.org/wp-content/uploads/2015/05/ICER_Preoperative-Stress-Testing.pdf.

19. Reed and Pearson, "Choosing Wisely® Recommendation Analysis."

20. Daniel Kahneman, *Thinking, Fast and Slow* (New York: Farrar, Straus and Giroux, 2013).

21. George A. Beller, "Tests that May Be Overused or Misused in Cardiology: The Choosing Wisely Campaign," *Journal of Nuclear Cardiology* 19, no.3 (2012): 401–403, https://link.springer.com/article/10.1007%2Fs12350-012-9569-y; American Board of Internal Medicine Foundation, "American College of Cardiology: Five Things Physicians and Patients Should Question," Choosing Wisely (website), updated February 28, 2017, http://www.choosingwisely.org/societies/american-college-of-cardiology/.

22. American Board of Internal Medicine Foundation, "American College of Cardiology."

23. Beller, "Tests that May Be Overused."

24. Lee A. Fleisher et al., "2014 ACC/AHA Guideline on Perioperative Cardiovascular Evaluation and Management of Patients Undergoing Noncardiac Surgery: A Report of the American College of Cardiology/American Heart Association Task Force on Practice Guidelines," *Journal of the American College of Cardiology* 64, no. 22 (2014): e77–137, http://www.onlinejacc.org/content/64/22/e77.

25. American Board of Internal Medicine Foundation, "American College of Cardiology"; Beller, "Tests that May Be Overused."

26. Jamieson M. Bourque et al., "Prognosis in Patients Achieving ≥ 10 METS on Exercise Stress Testing: Was SPECT Imaging Useful?" *Journal of Nuclear Cardiology* 18, no. 2 (2011): 230–37, https://www.ncbi.nlm.nih.gov/pmc/articles/PMC3902109/.

CHAPTER 2: CARDIAC CATHETERIZATION: THAT'S OUR PROTOCOL

1. Russell Lincoln Ackoff, *Redesigning the Future: A Systems Approach to Societal Problems* (New York: John Wiley and Sons, 1974), 8.

2. *Encyclopedia.com*, s.v. "Hales, Stephen," accessed July 3, 2018, https://www.encyclopedia.com/people/science-and-technology/biology-biographies/stephen-hales.

3. Heiss, H. W., and Hurst, J. Willis, "Werner forssmann: A german problem with the nobel prize." *Clinical Cardiology* 15 (7): 547–49 (1992).

4. Thirty years after his initial efforts, along with two American scientists, Werner was awarded the Nobel Prize in Medicine for his seminal work. Werner, by then an anonymous physician, remarked, "I feel like the village person who has just learned that he has been made bishop." *Encyclopedia.com*, s.v. "Hales, Stephen"; Ran Levi, "The Unbelievable Story behind the Invention of Cardiac Catheterization," *Medium* (website), February 17, 2016, https://medium.com/@ranlevi/the-unbelievable-story-behind-the-invention-of-cardiac-catheterization-ac09640cb92d.

5. Bousfield, "Angina Pectoris," 475; F. M. Smith "The Ligation of the Coronary Arteries with Electrocardiographic Study," *Archives of Internal Medicine* 22, no. 1 (1918): 8–27; Oppenheimer and Rothschild, "Electrocardiographic Changes Associated with Myocardial Involvement"; Pardee, "An Electrocardiographic Sign of Coronary Artery Obstruction."

6. Francis C. Wood and Charles C. Wolferth, "Angina Pectoris: The Clinical and Electrocardiographic Phenomena of the Attack and Their Comparison with the Effects

of Experimental Coronary Occlusion," *Archives of Internal Medicine* 47, no. 3 (1931): 339–65; Charles C. Wolferth, "The Diagnosis and Treatment of Acute Coronary Occlusion," *Medical Clinics of North America* 21, no. 4 (1937): 991–1001.

7. Thomas J. Ryan, "The Coronary Angiogram and Its Seminal Contributions to Cardiovascular Medicine Over Five Decades," *Circulation* 106, no. 6 (2002): 752–56, https://www.ahajournals.org/doi/full/10.1161/01.CIR.0000024109.12658.D4.

8. Ibid.; Albert V. G. Brushchke et al., "A Half Century of Selective Coronary Arteriography," *Journal of the American College of Cardiology* 54, no. 23 (2009): 2139–44, https://www.sciencedirect.com/science/article/pii/S0735109709030083?via%3Dihub.

9. Brushchke et al., "A Half Century of Selective Coronary Arteriography."

10. Ibid.

11. Ibid.

12. Steven J. Bernstein et al., "Coronary Angiography: A Literature Review and Ratings of Appropriateness and Necessity," Santa Monica, CA: RAND Corporation, 1992, available for download at https://www.rand.org/pubs/joint_reports-health/JRA03 .html; Dariush Mozaffarian et al., "Heart Disease and Stroke Statistics—2015 Update: A Report from the American Heart Association," *Circulation* 131, no. 4 (2015): e29–322, https://www.ahajournals.org/doi/full/10.1161/cir.0000000000000152.

13. F. L. Lucas et al., "Temporal Trends in the Utilization of Diagnostic Testing and Treatments for Cardiovascular Disease in the United States, 1993–2001," *Circulation* 113, no. 3 (2006): 374–79, https://www.ahajournals.org/doi/full/10.1161/CIRCULATION AHA.105.560433.

14. Manesh R. Patel et al., "Low Diagnostic Yield of Elective Coronary Angiography," *The New England Journal of Medicine* 362, no. 10 (2010): 886–95, https://www .nejm.org/doi/full/10.1056/NEJMoa0907272.

15. Ibid.

16. Steven M. Bradley et al., "Patient Selection for Diagnostic Coronary Angiography and Hospital-Level Percutaneous Coronary Intervention Appropriateness: Insights from the National Cardiovascular Data Registry," *JAMA Internal Medicine* 174, no.10 (2014): 1630–39, https://jamanetwork.com/journals/jamainternalmedicine/ fullarticle/1898877.

17. Edward L. Hannan et al., "Appropriateness of Diagnostic Catheterization for Suspected Coronary Artery Disease in New York State," *Circulation: Cardiovascular Interventions* 7, no. 1 (2014): 19–27, https://www.ahajournals.org/doi/10.1161/CIRC INTERVENTIONS.113.000741.

18. Bradley et al., "Patient Selection for Diagnostic Coronary Angiography."

19. Lucian L. Leape et al., "Effect of Variability in the Interpretation of Coronary Angiograms on the Appropriateness of Use of Coronary Revascularization Procedures," *American Heart Journal* 139, no. 1 (2000): 106–13, https://www.sciencedirect.com/ science/article/pii/S0002870300700160?via%3Dihub.

20. Patel et al., "Low Diagnostic Yield of Elective Coronary Angiography"; Nanette M. Borren et al., "Coronary Artery Stenoses More Often Overestimated in Older Patients: Angiographic Stenosis Overestimation in Elderly," *International Journal of Cardiology* 241 (2017): 46–49.

21. Therese A. Stukel, Lee F. Lucas, and David E. Wennberg, "Long-Term Outcomes of Regional Variations in Intensity of Invasive vs Medical Management of Medicare Patients with Acute Myocardial Infarction," *JAMA* 293, no. 11 (2005): 1329–37, https://jamanetwork.com/journals/jama/fullarticle/200542; Mudrick et al., "Patterns of Stress Testing and Diagnostic Catheterization."

22. American Heart Association, "Lifestyle Changes for Heart Attack Prevention."

23. Leape et al., "Effect of Variability in the Interpretation of Coronary Angiograms"; Stephan D. Fihn et al., "2012 ACCF / AHA / ACP / AATS / PCNA / SCAI / STS Guideline for the Diagnosis and Management of Patients with Stable Ischemic Heart Disease: Executive Summary," *Circulation* 126, no. 25 (2012): 3097–3137, https://www.ahajournals.org/doi/10.1161/CIR.0b013e3182776f83.

24. Borren et al., "Coronary Artery Stenoses More Often Overestimated in Older Patients"; Morteza Tavakol, Salman Ashraf, and Sorin J. Brener, "Risks and Complications of Coronary Angiography: A Comprehensive Review," *Global Journal of Health Science* 4, no.1 (2012): 65–93, https://www.ncbi.nlm.nih.gov/pmc/articles/PMC4777042/.

CHAPTER 3: ANGIOPLASTY: IT'S NOT KILLING YOU!

1. "I suppose it is tempting," wrote Abraham Maslow in 1966, "if the only tool you have is a hammer, to treat everything as if it were a nail." The popular aphorism has since been frequently borrowed and rephrased. Abraham H. Maslow, *The Psychology of Science: A Reconnaissance* (New York: Harper and Row, 1966), 15.

2. Matthias Barton et al., "Balloon Angioplasty—The Legacy of Andreas Grüntzig, M.D. (1939–1985)," *Frontiers in Cardiovascular Medicine* 1, no. 15 (2014), http://doi.org/10.3389/fcvm.2014.00015.

3. Geoffrey Rose, eulogizing fellow epidemiologist Donald Reid, as quoted in Henry Blackburn, "Donald Reid, MD," University of Minnesota (website), last modified October 15, 2012, http://www.epi.umn.edu/cvdepi/bio-sketch/reid-donald/.

4. Barton et al., "Balloon Angioplasty."

5. Spencer B. King III, "Angioplasty from Bench to Bedside to Bench," *Circulation* 93, no. 9 (1996): 1621–29, https://www.ahajournals.org/doi/10.1161/01.CIR.93.9.1621.

6. Ibid.

7. Barton et al., "Balloon Angioplasty."

8. Ibid.

9. Frederick A. Masoudi et al., "Trends in U.S. Cardiovascular Care: 2016 Report from 4 ACC National Cardiovascular Data Registries," *Journal of the American College of Cardiology* 69, no. 11 (2017): 1427–50, https://doi.org/10.1016/j.jacc.2016.12.005.

10. Kahneman, *Thinking, Fast and Slow*.

11. Tricia Bishop, "Mark Midei Fights for Medical License, Exoneration," *Baltimore Sun*, December 10, 2011, http://www.baltimoresun.com/health/bs-md-mark-midei-exclusive-20111210-story.html (accessed July 15, 2018).

12. Ibid.

13. Larry Husten, "Mark Midei Can't Get a Job Taking Blood Pressure at a Walmart," *Forbes*, April 8, 2012, https://www.forbes.com/sites/larryhusten/2012/04/08/mark -midei-cant-get-a-job-taking-blood-pressure-at-a-walmart/.

14. Bishop, "Mark Midei Fights for Medical License."

15. Tricia Bishop, "Federal Report on Stent Procedures Finds Potential Fraud," *Baltimore Sun*, December 6, 2010, http://articles.baltimoresun.com/2010-12-06/health/ bs-md-senate-stent-report-20101205_1_stent-procedures-midei-abbott-brand.

16. Ibid.; Advisory Board, "Behind Bars: The Downfall of the Nation's Busiest Cardiologist," October 31, 2013, https://www.advisory.com/Daily-Briefing/2013/10/31/ Behind-bars-The-downfall-of-the-nation-busiest-cardiologist; Joanna Walters, "Doctor Who Ordered Unnecessary Heart Surgery and Risky Tests Jailed for 20 Years," *The Guardian*, December 22 2015, https://www.theguardian.com/us-news/2015/dec/22/ doctor-who-ordered-unnecessary-heart-surgery-and-risky-tests-jailed-for-20-years.

17. Peter Waldman, David Armstrong, and Sydney P. Freedberg, "Deaths Linked to Cardiac Stents Rise as Overuse Seen," *Bloomberg News*, September 25, 2013, https:// www.bloomberg.com/news/articles/2013-09-26/deaths-linked-to-cardiac-stents-rise -as-overuse-seen.

18. Edward L. Hannan et al., "Appropriateness of Coronary Revascularization for Patients without Acute Coronary Syndromes," *Journal of the American College of Cardiology* 59, no. 21 (2012): 1870–76, http://www.onlinejacc.org/content/59/21/1870; Nihar R. Desai et al., "Appropriate Use Criteria for Coronary Revascularization and Trends in Utilization, Patient Selection, and Appropriateness of Percutaneous Coronary Intervention," *JAMA* 314, no. 19 (2015): 2045–53, https://jamanetwork.com/ journals/jama/fullarticle/2469192.

19. Waldman, Armstrong, and Freedberg, "Deaths Linked to Cardiac Stents."

20. The Dartmouth Atlas Project compiles searchable data about health-care practices across the United States. Visit their webpage at http://www.dartmouthatlas.org for more information on how medical resources are used nationally. Also see Michael P. Thomas et al., "Percutaneous Coronary Intervention Utilization and Appropriateness across the United States," *PLOS One* 10, no. 9 (2015): e0138251, https://doi .org/10.1371/journal.pone.0138251.

21. The NNT Group, "Stents for Stable Coronary Artery Disease," updated January 8, 2018, http://www.thennt.com/nnt/stents-stable-coronary-artery-disease/.

22. Anupam B. Jena et al., "Mortality and Treatment Patterns among Patients Hospitalized with Acute Cardiovascular Conditions during Dates of National Cardiology Meetings," *JAMA Internal Medicine* 175, no. 2 (2015): 237–44, https://jamanetwork .com/journals/jamainternalmedicine/fullarticle/2038979.

23. William B. Borden et al., "Patterns and Intensity of Medical Therapy in Patients Undergoing Percutaneous Coronary Intervention," *JAMA* 305, no. 18 (2011): 1882–89, https://jamanetwork.com/journals/jama/fullarticle/899881.

24. Waldman, Armstrong, and Freedberg, "Deaths Linked to Cardiac Stents."

25. Andrew J. Epstein et al., "Coronary Revascularization Trends in the United States, 2001–2008," *JAMA* 305, no. 17 (2011): 1769–76, https://jamanetwork.com/ journals/jama/fullarticle/899648.

26. Michael B. Rothberg et al., "Patients' and Cardiologists' Perceptions of the Benefits of Percutaneous Coronary Intervention for Stable Coronary Disease," *Annals of Internal Medicine* 153, no. 5 (2010): 307–13.

27. Michael B. Rothberg et al., "The Effect of Information Presentation on Beliefs about the Benefits of Elective Percutaneous Coronary Intervention," *JAMA Internal Medicine* 174, no. 10 (2014): 1623–29, https://jamanetwork.com/journals/jamainternal medicine/fullarticle/1898876.

28. Goff et al., "How Cardiologists Present the Benefits of Percutaneous Coronary Interventions."

29. Jonathan St. B. T. Evans, Stephen E. Newstead, and Ruth M. J. Byrne, *Human Reasoning: The Psychology of Deduction* (Hillsdale, NJ: Lawrence Erlbaum Associates, 1993).

30. Grace A. Lin, R. Adams Dudley, and Rita F. Redberg, "Cardiologists' Use of Percutaneous Coronary Interventions for Stable Coronary Artery Disease," *Archives of Internal Medicine* 167, no. 15 (2007): 1604–1609, https://jamanetwork.com/journals/jamainternalmedicine/fullarticle/769857.

31. Kathleen Stergiopoulos and David L. Brown, "Initial Coronary Stent Implantation with Medical Therapy vs Medical Therapy Alone for Stable Coronary Artery Disease: Meta-Analysis of Randomized Controlled Trials," *Archives of Internal Medicine* 172, no. 4 (2012): 312–29, https://jamanetwork.com/journals/jamainternalmedicine/fullarticle/1108733; David L. Brown and Rita F. Redberg, "Last Nail in the Coffin for PCI in Stable Angina?" *The Lancet* 391, no. 10115 (2018): 3–4; David L. Brown and Rita F. Redberg, "Continuing Use of Prophylactic Percutaneous Coronary Intervention in Patients with Stable Coronary Artery Disease Despite Evidence of No Benefit: Déjà Vu All Over Again," *JAMA Internal Medicine* 176, no. 5 (2016): 597–98; William E. Boden et al., "Optimal Medical Therapy with or without PCI for Stable Coronary Disease," *The New England Journal of Medicine* 356, no. 15 (2007): 1503–16, https://www.nejm.org/doi/full/10.1056/NEJMoa070829.

32. Paul S. Chan et al., "Patient and Hospital Characteristics Associated with Inappropriate Percutaneous Coronary Interventions," *Journal of the American College of Cardiology* 62, no. 24 (2013): 2274–81, https://doi.org/10.1016/j.jacc.2013.07.086.

33. Grace A. Lin, R. Adams Dudley, and Rita F. Redberg, "Why Physicians Favor Use of Percutaneous Coronary Intervention to Medical Therapy: A Focus Group Study," *Journal of General Internal Medicine* 23, no. 9 (2008): 1458–63, https://www.ncbi.nlm.nih.gov/pmc/articles/PMC2518034/.

34. Fihn et al., "2012 ACCF / AHA / ACP / AATS / PCNA / SCAI / STS Guideline."

35. Stergiopoulos and Brown, "Initial Coronary Stent Implantation"; Brown and Redberg, "Last Nail in the Coffin for PCI in Stable Angina?"; Boden et al., "Optimal Medical Therapy."

36. Fihn et al., "2012 ACCF / AHA / ACP / AATS / PCNA / SCAI / STS Guideline."

37. Stephen E. Kimmel, Jesse A. Berlin, Sean Hennessy, Brian L. Strom, Ronald J. Krone, and Warren K. Laskey for the Registry Committee of the Society for Cardiac

Angiography and Interventions, "Risk of Major Complications from Coronary Angio-plasty Performed Immediately after Diagnostic Coronary Angiography: Results from the Registry of the Society for Cardiac Angiography and Interventions," *Journal of the American College of Cardiology* 30, no. 1 (1997): 193–200, https://www.sciencedirect .com/science/article/pii/S0735109797001496.

CHAPTER 4: BYPASS SURGERY: A SECOND OPINION

1. *An Essay on Criticism* (London: Printed for W. Lewis in Russel Street, Covent Garden; and Sold by W. Taylor at the Ship in Pater-Noster Row, T. Osborn Near the Walks, and J. Graves in St. James Street, 1711), 36.

2. Wood and Wolferth, "Angina Pectoris."

3. *Wikipedia*, s.v. "Siege of Leningrad," last edited January 28, 2019, https:// en.wikipedia.org/wiki/Siege_of_Leningrad.

4. Igor E. Konstantinov, "Vasilii I Kolesov: A Surgeon to Remember," *Texas Heart Institute Journal* 31, no. 4 (2004): 349–58, https://www.ncbi.nlm.nih.gov/pmc/ articles/PMC548233/.

5. H. D. McIntosh and J. A. Garcia, "The First Decade of Aortocoronary Bypass Grafting, 1967–1977. A Review," *Circulation* 57, no. 3 (1978): 405–31, https://doi .org/10.1161/01.CIR.57.3.405; D. W. Miller et al., "The Practice of Coronary Artery Bypass Surgery in 1980," *Journal of Thoracic Cardiovascular Surgery* 81, no. 3 (1981): 423–27.

6. Epstein et al., "Coronary Revascularization Trends"; Yariv Gerber et al., "Coronary Revascularization in the Community: A Population-Based Study, 1990 to 2004," *Journal of the American College of Cardiology* 50, no. 13 (2007): 1223–29, https://doi .org/10.1016/j.jacc.2007.06.022; Richard F. Gillum, "Coronary Artery Bypass Surgery and Coronary Angiography in the United States, 1979–1983," *American Heart Journal* 113, no. 5 (1987): 1255–60.

7. Eugene Braunwald, "Coronary Artery Bypass Surgery—An Assessment," *Postgraduate Medical Journal* 52, no. 614 (1976): 733–38, https://pmj.bmj.com/content/ postgradmedj/52/614/733.full.pdf.

8. Stuart J. Head, Teresa M. Kieser, Volkmar Falk, Hans A. Huysmans, and A. Pieter Kappetein, "Coronary Artery Bypass Grafting: Part 1—The Evolution Over the First 50 Years," *European Heart Journal* 34, no. 37 (2013): 2862–72, https://doi .org/10.1093/eurheartj/eht330; Salim Yusuf et al., "Effect of Coronary Artery Bypass Graft Surgery on Survival: Overview of 10-Year Results from Randomised Trials by the Coronary Artery Bypass Graft Surgery Trialists Collaboration," *The Lancet* 344, no. 8922 (1994): 563–70.

9. Kurt Eichenwald, "Operating Profits: Mining Medicare; How One Hospital Benefited from Questionable Surgery," *New York Times*, August 12, 2003, https://www .nytimes.com/2003/08/12/business/operating-profits-mining-medicare-one-hospital -benefited-questionable-surgery.html.

10. Andrew Pollack, "California Patients Talk of Needless Heart Surgery," *New York Times*, November 4, 2002, https://www.nytimes.com/2002/11/04/business/california-patients-talk-of-needless-heart-surgery.html.

11. Sue Chan, "Surgery for Profit?" CBS News, November 21, 2002, https://www.cbsnews.com/news/surgery-for-profit/.

12. Pollack, "California Patients Talk of Needless Heart Surgery."

13. Stephen Klaidman, *Coronary: A True Story of Medicine Gone Awry* (New York: Scribner, 2007); Ryan Sabalow, "Moon Loses License" (*Redding, California*) *Record Searchlight*, November 14, 2007, http://archive.redding.com/news/moon-loses-license-ep-378302418-356395691.html/.

14. Rothberg et al., "Patients' and Cardiologists' Perceptions."

15. Goff et al., "How Cardiologists Present the Benefits."

16. The Dartmouth Atlas Project compiles searchable data about health-care practices across the United States. Visit their webpage at http://www.dartmouthatlas.org for more information on how medical resources are used nationally; Dartmouth Atlas Project, *Cardiac Surgery Report*, Dartmouth Atlas of Health Care: Studies of Surgical Variation, 2005, Center for the Evaluative Clinical Sciences, http://archive.dartmouthatlas.org/downloads/reports/Cardiac_report_2005.pdf.

17. Jack V. Tu et al., "Use of Cardiac Procedures and Outcomes in Elderly Patients with Myocardial Infarction in the United States and Canada," *The New England Journal of Medicine* 336, no. 21 (1997): 1500–1505, https://www.nejm.org/doi/full/10.1056/NEJM199705223362106.

18. Chad T. Wilson et al., "U.S. Trends in CABG Hospital Volume: The Effect of Adding Cardiac Surgery Programs," *Health Affairs* 26, no. 1 (2007): 162–68, https://doi.org/10.1377/hlthaff.26.1.162.

19. Wolters Kluwer, "Stable Ischemic Heart Disease: Overview of Care," *UpToDate* (website), last updated February 18, 2019, https://www.uptodate.com/contents/stable-ischemic-heart-disease-overview-of-care.

20. Ibid.

21. The NNT Group, "Coronary Artery Bypass Graft Surgery (Heart Bypass) for Preventing Death Over Ten Years," last updated July 20, 2014, http://www.thennt.com/nnt/coronary-heart-bypass-surgery-for-prevention-of-death/.

22. Wolters Kluwer, "Stable Ischemic Heart Disease: Indications for Revascularization," *UpToDate* (website), last updated February 18, 2019, https://www.uptodate.com/contents/stable-ischemic-heart-disease-indications-for-revascularization.

23. L. David Hillis et al., "2011 ACCF/AHA Guideline for Coronary Artery Bypass Graft Surgery: A Report of the American College of Cardiology Foundation/American Heart Association Task Force on Practice Guidelines," *Circulation* 124, no. 23 (2011): e652–e735, https://doi.org/10.1161/CIR.0b013e31823c074e.

24. Małgorzata Zalewska-Adamiec et al., "Prognosis in Patients with Left Main Coronary Artery Disease Managed Surgically, Percutaneously or Medically: A Long-Term Follow-Up," *Kardiologia Polska* 71, no. 8 (2013): 787–95, https://ojs.kardiologiapolska.pl/kp/article/view/KP.2013.0189/7409.

25. Masanori Fukunishi et al., "J-SAP Study 1–2: Outcomes of Patients with Stable High-Risk Coronary Artery Disease Receiving Medical-Preceding Therapy in Japan," *Circulation* 70, no. 8 (2006): 1012–16.

26. Find the Society of Thoracic Surgeons' Online STS Adult Cardiac Surgery Risk Calculator at http://riskcalc.sts.org/stswebriskcalc/calculate.

CHAPTER 5: SUPPLEMENTS, THE INTERNET, AND HEART MONITORS: THE CUSTOMER HAS THE CONTROLS

1. Robert G. Hart et al., "Antithrombotic Therapy to Prevent Stroke in Patients with Atrial Fibrillation: A Meta-Analysis," *Annals of Internal Medicine* 131, no. 7 (1999): 492–501, http://annals.org/aim/fullarticle/712970/therapy-prevent-stroke -patients-atrial-fibrillation.

2. Craig T. January et al., "2014 AHA/ACC/HRS Guideline for the Management of Patients with Atrial Fibrillation: Executive Summary," *Journal of the American College of Cardiology* 64, no. 21 (2014): 2246–80, http://www.onlinejacc.org/content/ 64/21/2246 http://www.onlinejacc.org/content/64/21/2246.

3. Visit the National Center for Complementary and Integrative Health online at https://nccih.nih.gov.

4. As quoted from the NCCIH website by Janet Helm, "Getting to the Root of the Turmeric Trend," *Nutrition Unplugged*, June 6, 2015, https://www.nutritionunplugged .com/2015/06/getting-root-turmeric-trend/.

5. Steven G. Newmaster et al., "DNA Barcoding Detects Contamination and Substitution in North American Herbal Products," *BMC Medicine* 11, no. 1 (2013): 222, https://doi.org/10.1186/1741-7015-11-222.

6. Chor Kwan Ching et al., "Adulteration of Herbal Antidiabetic Products with Undeclared Pharmaceuticals: A Case Series in Hong Kong," *British Journal of Clinical Pharmacology* 73, no. 5 (2012): 795–800, https://doi.org/10.1111/j.1365 -2125.2011.04135.x.

7. K. Aleisha Fetters, "6 Myths about Nutritional Supplements You Must Know," *U.S. News and World Report*, April 27, 2018, https://health.usnews.com/wellness/food/ articles/2018-04-27/6-myths-about-nutritional-supplements-you-must-know; US Food and Drug Administration, "FDA 101: Dietary Supplements," last updated November 6, 2017, https://www.fda.gov/ForConsumers/ConsumerUpdates/ucm050803.htm.

8. David M. Eisenberg et al., "Trends in Alternative Medicine Use in the United States, 1990–1997: Results of a Follow-Up National Survey," *JAMA* 280, no. 18 (1998): 1569–75, https://jamanetwork.com/journals/jama/fullarticle/188148; Market Research Future, "Future Trend of Herbal Medicine Market 2018 Scope | at a CAGR of ~7.2% during 2017 to 2023 | Increasing Demand for Safe Therapies," Reuters, April 12, 2018, https://www.reuters.com/brandfeatures/venture-capital/article?id=32992; Hexa Research, "Herbal Medicine Market Size and Forecast, by Product (Tablets and

Capsules, Powders, Extracts), by Indication (Digestive Disorders, Respiratory Disorders, Blood Disorders), and Trend Analysis, 2014–2024," September 2017, https://www.hexaresearch.com/research-report/global-herbal-medicine-market.

9. Rebecca J. Cohen, Kirsten Ek, and Cynthia X. Pan, "Complementary and Alternative Medicine (CAM) Use by Older Adults: A Comparison of Self-Report and Physician Chart Documentation," *The Journals of Gerontology: Series A* 57, no. 4 (2002): M223–27, https://doi.org/10.1093/gerona/57.4.M223.

10. Newmaster et al., "DNA Barcoding Detects Contamination and Substitution"; E. Ernst, "Adulteration of Chinese Herbal Medicines with Synthetic Drugs: A Systematic Review," *Journal of Internal Medicine* 252, no. 2 (2002): 107–13, https://doi.org/10.1046/j.1365-2796.2002.00999.x; Grace M. Kuo et al., "Factors Associated with Herbal Use among Urban Multiethnic Primary Care Patients: A Cross-Sectional Survey," *BMC Complementary and Alternative Medicine* 4 (2004): 18, https://doi.org/10.1186/1472-6882-4-18; Annette S. Gross et al., "Influence of Grapefruit Juice on Cisapride Pharmacokinetics," *Clinical Pharmacology and Therapeutics* 65, no. 4 (1999): 395–401; Ara Tachjian, Viqar Maria, and Arshad Jahangir, "Use of Herbal Products and Potential Interactions in Patients with Cardiovascular Diseases," *Journal of the American College of Cardiology* 55, no. 6 (2010): 515–25, https://www.ncbi.nlm.nih.gov/pmc/articles/PMC2831618/.

11. Andrew I. Geller et al., "Emergency Department Visits for Adverse Events Related to Dietary Supplements," *The New England Journal of Medicine* 373, no. 16 (2015): 1531–40, https://www.nejm.org/doi/full/10.1056/nejmsa1504267.

12. Victor J. Navarro et al., "Liver Injury from Herbals and Dietary Supplements in the U.S. Drug-Induced Liver Injury Network," *Hepatology* 60, no. 4 (2014): 1399–408, https://doi.org/10.1002/hep.27317.

13. Eisenberg et al., "Trends in Alternative Medicine Use.

14. US Food and Drug Administration, "Development and Approval Process (Drugs)," last updated June 13, 2018, https://www.fda.gov/drugs/developmentapprovalprocess/default.htm.

15. A number of reputable medical sources can be found online. Among them, find Mayo Clinic's Patient Care and Health Information portal at https://www.mayoclinic.org/patient-care-and-health-information. Cleveland Clinic offers an online Health Library at https://my.clevelandclinic.org/health. WebMD provides credible information on a variety of health topics at https://www.webmd.com. The American College of Cardiology's Patient Self Care Education (Outpatient Setting) online toolkit is available at https://www.acc.org/tools-and-practice-support/clinical-toolkits/heart-failure-practice-solutions/patient-self-care-education-outpatient-setting.

16. Jeongeun Kim and Sukwha Kim, "Physicians' Perception of the Effects of Internet Health Information on the Doctor–Patient Relationship," *Informatics for Health and Social Care* 34, no. 3 (2009): 136–48; *Glamour*, "Why You Should Never Google Your Symptoms," Well + Good, September 25, 2015, https://www.glamour.com/story/why-you-should-never-google-yo.

17. Hannah L. Semigran, David M. Levine, et al., "Comparison of Physician and Computer Diagnostic Accuracy," *JAMA Internal Medicine* 176 (12) (2016): 1860–61.

18. Gina Kolata, "'Maximum' Heart Rate Theory Is Challenged," *New York Times*, April 24, 2001, https://www.nytimes.com/2001/04/24/health/maximum-heart-rate -theory-is-challenged.html.

19. Ibid.

20. Ibid.

21. Benjamin Keller, "Self-Tracking, to the Point of Obsession," *In Vivo*, November 12, 2014, http://www.invivomagazine.com/en/corpore_sano/tendances/article/66/self -tracking-to-the-point-of-obsession.

22. Nick Bilton, "For Fitness Bands, Slick Marketing but Suspect Results," Bits, *New York Times*, April 27, 2014, https://bits.blogs.nytimes.com/2014/04/27/for -fitness-bands-slick-marketing-but-suspect-results/.

23. David Freeman, "The Truth about Heart Rate and Exercise," WebMD, October 23, 2009, https://www.webmd.com/fitness-exercise/features/the-truth-about-heart -rate-and-exercise#1.

24. Edward Doris, Iain Matthews, and Honey Thomas, "Heart Rate Monitors and Fitness Trackers: Friend or Foe?" *British Journal of Cardiology* 24 (2017): 137–41; Lisa Cadmus-Bertram et al., "The Accuracy of Heart Rate Monitoring by Some Wrist-Worn Activity Trackers," *Annals of Internal Medicine* 166, no. 8 (2017): 610–12.

25. Keller, "Self-Tracking, to the Point of Obsession."

26. Doris, Matthews, and Thomas, "Heart Rate Monitors and Fitness Trackers."

27. Freeman, "The Truth about Heart Rate and Exercise."

28. Ibid.

CHAPTER 6: PACEMAKERS: A SUREFIRE SPARK?

1. O. Aquilina, "A Brief History of Cardiac Pacing," *Images in Paediatric Cardiology* 8, no. 2 (2006): 17–81, https://www.ncbi.nlm.nih.gov/pmc/articles/PMC3232561/.

2. Ibid.

3. Barnafeder, "Wilson Greatbatch, Inventor of Implantable Pacemaker, Dies at 92," *New York Times*, September 28, 2011, https://www.nytimes.com/2011/09/28/ business/wilson-greatbatch-pacemaker-inventor-dies-at-92.html.

4. Aquilina, "A Brief History of Cardiac Pacing."

5. Joseph Radder, "Wilson Greatbatch: Man of the Millennium," *Living Prime Time*, December 1999, http://www.livingprimetime.com/AllCovers/dec1999/workdec 1999/wilson_greatbatch_man_of_the_mil.htm.

6. Aquilina, "A Brief History of Cardiac Pacing."

7. Barnafeder, "Wilson Greatbatch, Inventor of Implantable Pacemaker, Dies at 92."

8. Aquilina, "A Brief History of Cardiac Pacing."

9. Barnafeder, "Wilson Greatbatch, Inventor of Implantable Pacemaker, Dies at 92."

10. David E. Bush and Thomas E. Finucane, "Permanent Cardiac Pacemakers in the Elderly," *Journal of the American Geriatric Society* 42, no. 3 (1994): 326–34; CBS News, Associated Press, "15-Minute-Old Premature Newborn Receives Pacemaker,"

updated February 16, 2012, https://www.cbsnews.com/news/15-minute-old-premature
-newborn-receives-pacemaker/.

11. J. H. Bennekers, Rob van Mechelen, and A. Meijer, "Pacemaker Safety and Long-Distance Running," *Netherlands Heart Journal* 12, no. 10 (2004): 450–54, https://www.ncbi.nlm.nih.gov/pmc/articles/PMC2497157/pdf/Nheartj00109-0018.pdf.

12. Erik O. Udo et al., on behalf of FOLLOWPACE study, "Survival and Determinants of Survival in Bradycardia Pacemaker Recipients: A Nationwide Cohort Study," *European Heart Journal*, 34 no.1, (2013): 2617.

13. Pat Croskerry, "The Importance of Cognitive Errors in Diagnosis and Strategies to Minimize Them," *Academic Medicine* 78, no. 8 (2003): 775–80, https://journals.lww.com/academicmedicine/Fulltext/2003/08000/The_Importance_of_Cognitive_Errors_in_Diagnosis.3.aspx.

14. Aquilina, "A Brief History of Cardiac Pacing."

15. Ibid.; Kirk Jeffrey and Victor Parsonnet, "Cardiac Pacing, 1960–1985: A Quarter Century of Medical and Industrial Innovation," *Circulation* 97, no. 19 (1998): 1978–91.

16. Barnafeder, "Wilson Greatbatch, Inventor of Implantable Pacemaker, Dies at 92."

17. Katy Butler, "What Broke My Father's Heart," *New York Times Magazine*, June 18, 2010, https://www.nytimes.com/2010/06/20/magazine/20pacemaker-t.html.

18. Ibid.; Pierluigi Tricoci et al., "Scientific Evidence Underlying the ACC/AHA Clinical Practice Guidelines," *JAMA* 301, no. 8 (2009): 831–41, https://jamanetwork.com/journals/jama/fullarticle/183453; Mark D. Neuman et al., "Durability of Class I American College of Cardiology/American Heart Association Clinical Practice Guideline Recommendations," *JAMA* 311, no. 20 (2014): 2092–100, https://jamanetwork.com/journals/jama/fullarticle/1874510; Terrence M. Shaneyfelt and Robert M. Centor, "Reassessment of Clinical Practice Guidelines: Go Gently into That Good Night," *JAMA* 301, no.8 (2009): 868–69.

19. Peter Eisler and Barbara Hansen, "Doctors Perform Thousands of Unnecessary Surgeries," *USA Today*, updated June 20, 2013, https://www.usatoday.com/story/news/nation/2013/06/18/unnecessary-surgery-usa-today-investigation/2435009/.

20. Brockton J. Hefflin, "Final-Year-of-Life Pacemaker Recipients," *Journal of the American Geriatrics Society* 46, no.11 (1998): 1396–400.

21. Allan M. Greenspan et al., "Incidence of Unwarranted Implantation of Permanent Cardiac Pacemakers in a Large Medical Population," *The New England Journal of Medicine* 318, no. 3 (1988): 158–63.

22. A. Greenberg et al., "Permanent Pacemakers in Maryland," report, Washington, DC: Health Research Group, 1982; Peter Russell Kowey et al., "State of Maryland Pacemaker Experience (1979–1980): Conflicting Views regarding the Frequency of Unnecessary Pacemaker Implants," *The American Journal of Cardiology* 51, no. 6 (1983): 1042–43; Martino Martinelli et al., "Criteria for Pacemaker Explant in Patients without a Precise Indication for Pacemaker Implantation," *Pacing and Clinical Electrophysiology* 25, no. 3 (2002): 272–77.

23. Muhammad Rizwan Sohail et al., "Infective Endocarditis Complicating Permanent Pacemaker and Implantable Cardioverter-Defibrillator Infection," *Mayo Clinic Proceedings* 83, no. 1 (2008): 46–53.

24. US Attorney's Office, Eastern District of Kentucky, "London Cardiologist Convicted of Health Care Fraud for Medically Unnecessary Pacemakers," US Department of Justice (website), April 16, 2018, https://www.justice.gov/usao-edky/pr/london -cardiologist-convicted-health-care-fraud-medically-unnecessary-pacemakers.

25. Ádám Böhm, Ferenc Bányai, István Préda, and Károly Zámolyi, "The Treatment of Septicemia in Pacemaker Patients," *Pacing and Clinical Electrophysiology* 19, no. 7 (1996): 1105–11; Charles L. Byrd et al., "Intravascular Extraction of Problematic or Infected Permanent Pacemaker Leads: 1994–1996. U.S. Extraction Database, MED Institute," *Pacing and Clinical Electrophysiology* 22, no. 9 (1999): 1348–57; William H. Maisel et al., "Recalls and Safety Alerts Involving Pacemakers and Implantable Cardioverter-Defibrillator Generators," *JAMA* 286, no. 7 (2001): 793–99, https://jamanetwork.com/journals/jama/fullarticle/194108; Chikashi Suga et al., "Is There an Adverse Outcome from Abandoned Pacing Leads?" *Journal of Interventional Cardiac Electrophysiology* 4, no. 3 (2000): 493–99; J. G. Voet et al., "Pacemaker Lead Infection: Report of Three Cases and Review of the Literature," *Heart* 81, no. 1 (1999): 88–91, http://dx.doi.org/10.1136/hrt.81.1.88; "Complications of Permanent Cardiac Pacemakers," letter to the editor, *The New England Journal of Medicine* 313, no. 17 (1985): 1085–88.

26. Fred M. Kusumoto et al., "2018 ACC/AHA/HRS Guideline on the Evaluation and Management of Patients with Bradycardia and Cardiac Conduction Delay," *Journal of the American College of Cardiology* (2018), https://doi.org/10.1016/j .jacc.2018.10.043.

27. National Heart, Lung, and Blood Institute, "Pacemakers," Health Topics, National Institute of Health (website), https://www.nhlbi.nih.gov/health-topics/pacemakers (accessed August 25, 2018).

28. Kusumoto et al., "2018 ACC/AHA/HRS Guideline."

29. "Complications of Permanent Cardiac pacemakers," *The New England Journal of Medicine.*

30. National Heart, Lung, and Blood Institute, "Pacemakers."

CHAPTER 7: DEFIBRILLATOR: MANY GET IT, SOME NEED IT

1. As quoted in Darren Dalcher, *Further Advances in Project Management: Guided Exploration in Unfamiliar Landscapes* (London: Routledge, 2016), 205.

2. Paul M. Zoll et al., "Termination of Ventricular Fibrillation in Man by Externally Applied Electric Countershock," *The New England Journal of Medicine* 254, no. 16 (1956): 727–32.

3. *Wikipedia*, s.v. "Michel Mirowski: Medical Training," last updated December 18, 2018, https://en.wikipedia.org/wiki/Michel_Mirowski#Medical_training; Marc W. Deyell, Stanley Tung, and Adrew Ignaszewski, "The Implantable Cardioverter-Defibrillator: From Mirowski to Its Current Use," *BC Medical Journal* 52, no. 5

(2010): 248–53, https://www.bcmj.org/articles/implantable-cardioverter-defibrillator-mirowski-its-current-use.

4. Deyell, Tung, and Ignaszewski, "The Implantable Cardioverter-Defibrillator."

5. Bernard Lown and Paul Axelrod, "Implanted Standby Defibrillators," *Circulation* 46, no. 4 (1972): 637–39, https://www.ahajournals.org/doi/pdf/10.1161/01.CIR.46.4.637, emphasis mine.

6. Zoll et al., "Termination of Ventricular Fibrillation."

7. Antiarrhythmics Versus Implantable Defibrillators (AVID) Investigators, "A Comparison of Antiarrhythmic-Drug Therapy with Implantable Defibrillators in Patients Resuscitated from Near-Fatal Ventricular Arrhythmias," *The New England Journal of Medicine* 337, no. 22 (1997): 1576–83, https://www.nejm.org/doi/10.1056/NEJM199711273372202.

8. Alfred E. Buxton et al., "A Randomized Study of the Prevention of Sudden Death in Patients with Coronary Artery Disease. Multicenter Unsustained Tachycardia Trial Investigators," *The New England Journal of Medicine* 341, no. 25 (1999): 1882–90, https://www.nejm.org/doi/10.1056/NEJM199912163412503; Arthur J. Moss et al., "Improved Survival with an Implanted Defibrillator in Patients with Coronary Disease at High Risk for Ventricular Arrhythmia. Multicenter Automatic Defibrillator Implantation Trial Investigators," *The New England Journal of Medicine* 335, no. 26 (1996): 1933–40, https://www.nejm.org/doi/10.1056/NEJM199612263352601; Gust H. Bardy et al., for the Sudden Cardiac Death in Heart Failure Trial (SCD-HeFT) Investigators, "Amiodarone or an Implantable Cardioverter-Defibrillator for Congestive Heart Failure," *The New England Journal of Medicine* 352, no. 3 (2005): 225–37, https://www.nejm.org/doi/full/10.1056/nejmoa043399.

9. Douglas P. Zipes et al., "ACC/AHA/ESC 2006 Guidelines for Management of Patients with Ventricular Arrhythmias and the Prevention of Sudden Cardiac Death—Executive Summary: A Report of the American College of Cardiology/American Heart Association Task Force and the European Society of Cardiology Committee for Practice Guidelines (Writing Committee to Develop Guidelines for Management of Patients with Ventricular Arrhythmias and the Prevention of Sudden Cardiac Death," *European Heart Journal* 114, no. 10 (2006): 1088–132, https://www.ahajournals.org/doi/pdf/10.1161/CIRCULATIONAHA.106.178104.

10. Antiarrhythmics . . . Investigators, "A Comparison of Antiarrhythmic-Drug Therapy"; Buxton et al., "A Randomized Study"; Moss et al., "Improved Survival with an Implanted Defibrillator"; Bardy et al., "Amiodarone or an Implantable Cardioverter-Defibrillator"; Zipes et al., "ACC/AHA/ESC 2006 Guidelines"; Timothy R. Betts et al., "Absolute Risk Reduction in Total Mortality with Implantable Cardioverter Defibrillators: Analysis of Primary and Secondary Prevention Trial Data to Aid Risk/Benefit Analysis," *EP Europace* 15, no. 6 (2013): 813–19, https://doi.org/10.1093/europace/eus427.

11. Medtronic, *Implantable Cardioverter-Defibrillators (ICDs)*, 2015, https://www.medtronic.com/content/dam/medtronic-com/us-en/newsroom/media-resources/media-kits/implantable-cardioverter-defibrillators/documents/icd-backgrounder-2015.pdf.

12. Harvard Health Publishing, "Shocking News: Overdoing ICDs," *Harvard Health Letter*, March 2011, https://www.health.harvard.edu/heart-health/shocking-news-overdoing-icds (subscription required).

13. Sana M. Al-Khatib et al., "Non-Evidence-Based ICD Implantations in the United States," *JAMA* 305, no. 1 (2011): 43–49, https://jamanetwork.com/journals/jama/fullarticle/644551.

14. Daniel D. Matlock et al., "Regional Variation in the Use of Implantable Cardioverter-Defibrillators for Primary Prevention: Results from the National Cardiovascular Data Registry," *Circulation. Cardiovascular Quality and Outcomes* 4, no. 1 (2011): 114–21, https://www.ahajournals.org/doi/10.1161/CIRCOUTCOMES.110.958264.

15. Zipes et al., "ACC/AHA/ESC 2006 Guidelines."

16. Al-Khatib et al., "Non-Evidence-Based ICD Implantations."

17. Lynne Warner Stevenson and Akshay S. Desai, "Selecting Patients for Discussion of the ICD as Primary Prevention for Sudden Death in Heart Failure," *Journal of Cardiac Failure* 12, no. 6 (2006): 407–12; Sérgio Barra et al., "Implantable Cardioverter-Defibrillators in the Elderly: Rationale and Specific Age-Related Considerations," *EP Europace* 17, no. 2 (2015): 174–86, https://doi.org/10.1093/europace/euu296; Andrew D. Krahn et al., "Diminishing Proportional Risk of Sudden Death with Advancing Age: Implications for Prevention of Sudden Death," *American Heart Journal* 147, no. 5 (2004): 837–40.

18. Michael Bar-Eli et al., "Action Bias among Elite Soccer Goalkeepers: The Case of Penalty Kicks," *Journal of Economic Psychology* 28, no. 5 (2007): 606–21.

19. Al-Khatib et al., "Non-Evidence-Based ICD Implantations."

20. Johannes B. van Rees et al., "Inappropriate Implantable Cardioverter-Defibrillator Shocks: Incidence, Predictors, and Impact on Mortality," *Journal of the American College of Cardiology* 57, no. 5 (2011): 556–62, https://doi.org/10.1016/j.jacc.2010.06.059; Jeanne E. Poole et al., "Prognostic Importance of Defibrillator Shocks in Patients with Heart Failure," *The New England Journal of Medicine* 359, no. 10 (2008): 1009–17, https://www.nejm.org/doi/full/10.1056/NEJMoa071098.

21. Samuel F. Sears et al., "Posttraumatic Stress and the Implantable Cardioverter-Defibrillator Patient: What the Electrophysiologist Needs to Know," *Circulation: Arrhythmia and Electrophysiology* 4, no. 2 (2011): 242–50, https://doi.org/10.1161/CIRCEP.110.957670; Gregory M. Marcus, Derrick W. Chan, and Rita F. Redberg, "Recollection of Pain Due to Inappropriate versus Appropriate Implantable Cardioverter-Defibrillator Shocks," *Pacing and Clinical Electrophysiology* 34, no. 3 (2011): 348–53.

22. Isuru Ranasinghe et al., "Long-Term Risk for Device-Related Complications and Reoperations after Implantable Cardioverter-Defibrillator Implantation: An Observational Cohort Study," *Annals of Internal Medicine* 165, no. 1 (2016): 20–29; Konstantinos A. Polyzos, Athanasios A. Konstantelias, and Matthew E. Falgas, "Risk Factors for Cardiac Implantable Electronic Device Infection: A Systematic Review and Meta-Analysis," *EP Europace* 17, no. 5 (2015): 767–77, https://doi.org/10.1093/europace/euv053.

23. Victor Parsonnet and Jerzy O. Giedwoyn, "Pacemaker Failure Following External Defibrillation" and author reply, *Circulation* 45, no. 5 (1972): 1144–45, https://www.ahajournals.org/doi/pdf/10.1161/01.CIR.45.5.1144-a.

24. US Department of Justice Office of Public Affairs, "Medical Device Manufacturer Guidant Sentenced for Failure to Report Defibrillator Safety Problems to FDA: Boston Scientific Subsidiary Sentenced to Pay Criminal Penalty of More than $296 Million and Three Years Probation," Justice News, US Department of Justice (website), updated September 15, 2014, https://www.justice.gov/opa/pr/medical -device-manufacturer-guidant-sentenced-failure-report-defibrillator-safety-problems.

25. US Department of Justice Office of Public Affairs, "Nearly 500 Hospitals Pay United States More than $250 Million to Resolve False Claims Act Allegations Related to Implantation of Cardiac Devices," Justice News, US Department of Justice (website), updated April 28, 2017, https://www.justice.gov/opa/pr/nearly-500-hospitals -pay-united-states-more-250-million-resolve-false-claims-act-allegations.

26. Ibid.

27. John Lynn Jefferies and Jeffrey A. Towbin, "Dilated Cardiomyopathy," *Lancet* 375, no. 9716 (2010): 752–62.

28. Mayo Clinic Staff, "Ventricular Tachycardia," Mayo Clinic (website), October 4, 2018, https://www.mayoclinic.org/diseases-conditions/ventricular-tachycardia/symptoms-causes/syc-20355138.

29. American Heart Association, "Implantable Cardioverter Defibrillator (ICD)," Heart.org, last reviewed September 30, 2016, http://www.heart.org/en/health -topics/arrhythmia/prevention—treatment-of-arrhythmia/implantable-cardioverter -defibrillator-icd.

30. Zipes et al., "ACC/AHA/ESC 2006 Guidelines."

31. Ibid.

32. Stevenson and Desai, "Selecting Patients for Discussion of the ICD."

33. Antiarrhythmics . . . Investigators, "A Comparison of Antiarrhythmic-Drug Therapy"; Buxton et al., "A Randomized Study"; Moss et al., "Improved Survival with an Implanted Defibrillator"; Bardy et al., "Amiodarone or an Implantable Cardioverter-Defibrillator"; Zipes et al., "ACC/AHA/ESC 2006 Guidelines."

34. Antiarrhythmics . . . Investigators, "A Comparison of Antiarrhythmic-Drug Therapy"; Buxton et al., "A Randomized Study"; Moss et al., "Improved Survival with an Implanted Defibrillator"; Zipes et al., "ACC/AHA/ESC 2006 Guidelines."

35. Ibid.

CHAPTER 8: ABLATION: CURING YOUR RHYTHM PROBLEMS

1. Hein J. J. Wellens, "Cardiac Arrhythmias: The Quest for a Cure; A Historical Perspective," *Journal of the American College of Cardiology* 44, no. 6 (2004): 1155–63, https://doi.org/10.1016/j.jacc.2004.05.080; J. P. Joseph and K. Rajappan, "Radiofre-

quency Ablation of Cardiac Arrhythmias: Past, Present and Future," *QJM* 105, no. 4 (2012): 303–14, https://doi.org/10.1093/qjmed/hcr189; Berndt Lüderitz, "Historical Perspectives on Interventional Electrophysiology," *Journal of Interventional Cardiac Electrophysiology* 9, no. 2 (2003): 75–83.

2. Wellens, "Cardiac Arrhythmias"; Joseph and Rajappan, "Radiofrequency Ablation"; Lüderitz, "Historical Perspectives."

3. Rolando Gonzalez et al., "Closed-Chest Electrode-Catheter Technique for His Bundle Ablation in Dogs," *American Journal of Physiology* 241, no. 2 (1981): H283–87; Melvin [M.] Scheinman and John D. Rutherford, "The Development of Cardiac Arrhythmia Ablation: A Conversation with Melvin A. Scheinman, MD," *Circulation* 135, no. 13 (2017): 1191–93, https://doi.org/10.1161/CIRCULATION AHA.117.027956; Melvin M. Scheinman et al., "Catheter-Induced Ablation of the Atrioventricular Junction to Control Refractory Supraventricular Arrhythmias," *JAMA* 248, no. 7 (1982): 851–55.

4. Marion A. Lee et al., "Catheter Modification of the Atrioventricular Junction with Radiofrequency Energy for Control of Atrioventricular Nodal Reentry Tachycardia," *Circulation* 83, no. 3 (1991): 827–35; Fred Morady and Melvin M. [Scheinman], "Transvenous Catheter Ablation of a Posteroseptal Accessory Pathway in a Patient with the Wolff-Parkinson-White Syndrome," *The New England Journal of Medicine* 310 (1984): 705–707; Fred Morady, "Catheter Ablation of Supraventricular Arrhythmias: State of the Art," *Pacing and Clinical Electrophysiology* 27, no. 1 (2004): 125–42.

5. John McMichael, "History of Atrial Fibrillation 1628–1819: Harvey–de Senac – Laënnec," *British Heart Journal* 48, no. 3 (1982): 193–97, https://www.ncbi.nlm .nih.gov/pmc/articles/PMC481228/; Gregory Y. H. Lip and D. Gareth Beevers, "ABC of Atrial Fibrillation: History, Epidemiology, and Importance of Atrial Fibrillation," *British Medical Journal* 311, no. 7016 (1995): 1361–63.

6. Philip A. Wolf et al., "Epidemiologic Assessment of Chronic Atrial Fibrillation and Risk of Stroke: The Framingham Study," *Neurology* 28, no. 10 (1978): 973–77.

7. Hart et al., "Antithrombotic Therapy."

8. Michel Haïssaguerre et al., "Spontaneous Initiation of Atrial Fibrillation by Ectopic Beats Originating in the Pulmonary Veins," *The New England Journal of Medicine* 339, no. 10 (1998): 659–66, https://www.nejm.org/doi/full/10.1056/ NEJM199809033391003.

9. Matteo Anselmino et al., "History of Transcatheter Atrial Fibrillation Ablation," *Journal of Cardiovascular Medicine* 13, no. 1 (2012): 1–8.

10. Centers for Disease Control and Prevention, "Atrial Fibrillation Fact Sheet," CDC.gov, last reviewed August 22, 2017, https://www.cdc.gov/dhdsp/data_statistics/ fact_sheets/fs_atrial_fibrillation.htm.

11. Consider the sheer proliferation of related professional conferences advertised at OMICS International, "Atrial Fibrillation," Conferences, https://www.omicsonline .org/conferences-list/atrial-fibrillation (accessed August 25, 2018).

12. Personal communication to the author, 2012.

13. Michael H. Kim et al., "Estimation of Total Incremental Health Care Costs in Patients with Atrial Fibrillation in the United States," *Circulation: Cardiovascular*

Quality Outcomes 4, no. 3 (2011): 313–20, https://doi.org/10.1161/CIRCOUTCOMES .110.958165; Shlomo Ben-Haim, "How Innovation Can Unleash Tremendous Growth in the $3.4 Billion AF Ablation Market," *Cardiac Rhythm News*, February 29, 216, https://cardiacrhythmnews.com/how-innovation-can-unleash-tremendous-growth-in-the -3-4-billion-af-ablation-market/.

14. Emelia J. Benjamin et al., "Impact of Atrial Fibrillation on the Risk of Death: The Framingham Heart Study," *Circulation* 98, no. 10 (1998): 946–52.

15. Simon Stewart et al., "Population Prevalence, Incidence, and Predictors of Atrial Fibrillation in the Renfrew/Paisley Study," *Heart* 86, no. 5 (2001): 516–21, http:// dx.doi.org/10.1136/heart.86.5.516; Wendy A. Wattigney, George A. Mensah, and Janet B. Croft, "Increased Atrial Fibrillation Mortality: United States, 1980–1998," *American Journal of Epidemiology* 155, no. 9 (2002): 819–26, https://doi.org/10.1093/ aje/155.9.819.

16. Valentin Fuster et al., "2011 ACCF/AHA/HRS Focused Updates Incorporated into the ACC/AHA/ESC 2006 Guidelines for the Management of Patients with Atrial Fibrillation: A Report of the American College of Cardiology Foundation/American Heart Association Task Force on Practice Guidelines," *Circulation* 123, no. 10 (2011): e269–367, https://doi.org/10.1161/CIR.0b013e318214876d.

17. D. George Wyse et al., "A Comparison of Rate Control and Rhythm Control in Patients with Atrial Fibrillation," *The New England Journal of Medicine* 347, no. 23 (2002): 1825–33, https://www.nejm.org/doi/full/10.1056/NEJMoa021328.

18. Isabelle C. Van Gelder et al., "A Comparison of Rate Control and Rhythm Control in Patients with Recurrent Persistent Atrial Fibrillation," *The New England Journal of Medicine* 347, no. 23 (2002): 1834–40, https://www.nejm.org/doi/full/10.1056/ NEJMoa021375.

19. A. John Camm et al., "Real-Life Observations of Clinical Outcomes with Rhythm- and Rate-Control Therapies for Atrial Fibrillation: RECORDAF (Registry on Cardiac Rhythm Disorders Assessing the Control of Atrial Fibrillation)," *Journal of the American College of Cardiology* 58, no. 5 (2011): 493–501, http://www.onlinejacc .org/content/58/5/493.full.

20. Daniel Caldeira, Cláudio David, and Cristina Sampaio, "Rate vs Rhythm Control in Patients with Atrial Fibrillation and Heart Failure: A Systematic Review and Meta-Analysis of Randomised Controlled Trials," *European Journal of Internal Medicine* 22, no. 5 (2011): 448–55.

21. Amit Noheria et al., "Rhythm Control versus Rate Control and Clinical Outcomes in Patients with Atrial Fibrillation: Results from the ORBIT-AF Registry," *JACC: Clinical Electrophysiology* 2, no. 2 (2016): 221–29, https://doi.org/10.1016/j .jacep.2015.11.001.

22. Abhishek Deshmukh et al., "In-Hospital Complications Associated with Catheter Ablation of Atrial Fibrillation in the United States between 2000 and 2010: Analysis of 93 801 Procedures," *Circulation* 128, no. 19 (2013): 2104–12, https:// doi.org/10.1161/CIRCULATIONAHA.113.003862; Richard J. Schilling and Razeen Gopal, "Mortality and Catheter Ablation of Atrial Fibrillation," *British Journal of*

Cardiology 17 (2010): 161–62, https://bjcardio.co.uk/2010/07/mortality-and-catheter-ablation-of-atrial-fibrillation/.

23. John Mandrola, "AF Ablation Is Overused in the US," *Dr. John M* (website), March 11, 2017, http://www.drjohnm.org/2017/03/af-ablation-is-overused-in-the-us/.

24. Douglas L. Packer et al., "Catheter Ablation versus Antiarrhythmic Drug Therapy for Atrial Fibrillation (CABANA) Trial: Study Rationale and Design," *American Heart Journal* 199 (2018): 192–99, https://doi.org/10.1016/j.ahj.2018.02.015.

25. American Heart Association, "What Is Arrhythmia?" 2015, https://www.heart.org/-/media/data-import/downloadables/pe-abh-what-is-arrhythmia-ucm_300290.pdf.

26. American Heart Association, "Tachycardia: Fast Heart Rate," Heart.org, last reviewed September 30, 2016, http://www.heart.org/en/health-topics/arrhythmia/about-arrhythmia/tachycardia—fast-heart-rate.

27. Ibid.

28. American Heart Association, "Ablation for Arrhythmias," Heart.org, last reviewed September 30, 2016, https://www.heart.org/en/health-topics/arrhythmia/prevention—treatment-of-arrhythmia/ablation-for-arrhythmias.

29. American Heart Association, "What Is Arrhythmia?"

30. Leonard I. Ganz, "Overview of Catheter Ablation of Cardiac Arrhythmias," *UpToDate*, Wolters Kluwer, last updated January 24, 2019, https://www.uptodate.com/contents/overview-of-catheter-ablation-of-cardiac-arrhythmias (subscription required).

31. Centers for Disease Control and Prevention, "Atrial Fibrillation Fact Sheet."

32. Ibid.

33. Ganz, "Overview of Catheter Ablation."

34. Centers for Disease Control and Prevention, "Atrial Fibrillation Fact Sheet."

35. Ganz, "Overview of Catheter Ablation."

36. American Heart Association, "What Is Arrhythmia?"

37. Laurent M. Haegli and Hugh Calkins, "Catheter Ablation of Atrial Fibrillation: An Update," *European Heart Journal* 35, no. 36 (2014): 2454–59, https://doi.org/10.1093/eurheartj/ehu291.

38. Deshmukh et al., "In-Hospital Complications."

39. Ganz, "Overview of Catheter Ablation."

CHAPTER 9: THE WAY FORWARD: THE HOME-CARE SOLUTION TO HEALTH CARE

1. Visit the National Center for Complementary and Integrative Health's website at https://nccih.nih.gov for a trustworthy source on unconventional medicine and the science behind health research.

2. Philip P. Goodney et al., "Consistency of Hemoglobin A1c Testing and Cardiovascular Outcomes in Medicare Patients with Diabetes," *Journal of the American Heart*

Association 5, no. 8 (2016): e003566, https://www.ncbi.nlm.nih.gov/pmc/articles/PMC5015285/.

3. Emanuel, "Are Good Doctors Bad for Your Health?"

4. Todd D. Miller, Rita F. Redberg, and Frans J. T. Wackers, "Screening Asymptomatic Diabetic Patients for Coronary Artery Disease: Why Not?" *Journal of the American College of Cardiology* 48, no. 4 (2006): 761–64, https://doi.org/10.1016/j.jacc.2006.04.076; David E. Wennberg et al., "The Association between Local Diagnostic Testing Intensity and Invasive Cardiac Procedures," *JAMA* 275, no. 15 (1996): 1161–64.

5. Roni Caryn Rabin, "Can You Miss the Signs of Heart Disease or a Heart Attack?" *New York Times*, April 20, 2018, https://www.nytimes.com/2018/04/20/well/live/signs-symptoms-heart-disease-heart-attack.html.

6. Diana Verrilli and H. Gilbert Welch, "The Impact of Diagnostic Testing on Therapeutic Interventions," *JAMA* 275, no.15 (1996): 1189–91.

7. Kathleen M. Fairfield et al., "Behavioral Risk Factors and Regional Variation in Cardiovascular Health Care and Death," *American Journal of Preventive Medicine* 54, no. 3 (2018): 376–84.

8. Aseem Malhotra, Rita F. Redberg, and Pascal Meier, "Saturated Fat Does Not Clog the Arteries: Coronary Heart Disease Is a Chronic Inflammatory Condition, the Risk of Which Can Be Effectively Reduced from Healthy Lifestyle Interventions," *British Journal of Sports Medicine* 51, no. 15 (2017): 1111–12, http://dx.doi.org/10.1136/bjsports-2016-097285.

9. H. Gilbert Welch, "If You Feel O.K., Maybe You Are O.K.," *New York Times*, February 27, 2012, https://www.nytimes.com/2012/02/28/opinion/overdiagnosis-as-a-flaw-in-health-care.html; Rita F. Redberg, "Talking about Patient Preferences," *JAMA Internal Medicine* 174, no. 3 (2014): 321, https://jamanetwork.com/journals/jamainternalmedicine/fullarticle/1809975.

10. For evidence-based advice on patient-led health care, visit Choosing Wisely, the American Board of Internal Medicine's Patient Resources portal, at http://www.choosingwisely.org/patient-resources/.

11. Gilbert, "If You Feel O.K., Maybe You Are O.K."; Redberg, "Talking about Patient Preferences."

12. The NNT Group provides an online resource for determining evidence-based medical care at http://www.thennt.com.

13. For more information on heart-healthy living, visit the American Heart Association's Healthy for Good website at https://www.heart.org/en/healthy-living.

14. Fairfield et al., "Behavioral Risk Factors."

15. Miller, Redberg, and Wackers, "Screening Asymptomatic Diabetic Patients"; Wennberg et al., "The Association between Local Diagnostic Testing Intensity"; Verrilli and Welch, "The Impact of Diagnostic Testing"; Malhotra, Redberg, and Meier, "Saturated Fat Does Not Clog the Arteries"; Laura Dwyer-Lindgren et al., "Inequalities in Life Expectancy among US Counties, 1980 to 2014: Temporal Trends and Key Drivers," *JAMA Internal Medicine* 177, no. 7 (2017): 1003–11, https://jamanetwork

.com/journals/jamainternalmedicine/fullarticle/2626194; American Heart Association, "Lifestyle Changes for Heart Attack Prevention."

16. Bourque et al,. "Prognosis in Patients."

17. Redberg, "Talking about Patient Preferences."

EPILOGUE: HEART-TO-HEART

1. Albert Schweitzer, *Kulturphilosophie* (Bern: P. Haupt, 1923), later translated into English by C. T. Campion as *Philosophy of Civilisation* (London: Black, 1932).

2. Kahneman, *Thinking, Fast and Slow*; Croskerry, "The Importance of Cognitive Errors in Diagnosis"; Jerome Groopman, *How Doctors Think* (Boston: Mariner Books, 2008); Bar-Eli et al., "Action Bias among Elite Soccer Goalkeepers"; Evans, Newstead, and Byrne, *Human Reasoning*.

3. Croskerry, "The Importance of Cognitive Errors in Diagnosis."

4. Kahneman, *Thinking, Fast and Slow*; Groopman, *How Doctors Think*.

5. Croskerry, "The Importance of Cognitive Errors in Diagnosis."

6. Bar-Eli et al., "Action Bias among Elite Soccer Goalkeepers."

7. Kahneman, *Thinking, Fast and Slow*; Groopman, *How Doctors Think*; Bar-Eli et al., "Action Bias among Elite Soccer Goalkeepers."

8. Croskerry, "The Importance of Cognitive Errors in Diagnosis."; Evans, Newstead, and Byrne, *Human Reasoning*.

9. Upton Sinclair, *I, Candidate for Governor: And How I Got Licked* (Pasadena, CA: Author, 1935).

10. Jacquelyn Smith, "The Best- And Worst-Paying Jobs for Doctors," *Forbes*, July 20, 2012, https://www.forbes.com/sites/jacquelynsmith/2012/07/20/the-best-and-worst-paying-jobs-for-doctors-2/#1c557431a2a3.

11. Marloes A. van Bokhoven et al., "Why Do Patients Want to Have Their Blood Tested? A Qualitative Study of Patient Expectations in General Practice," *BMC Family Practice* 7 (2006): 75–75, https://doi.org/10.1186/1471-2296-7-75.

12. Rainer S. Beck, Rebecca Daughtridge, and Philip D. Sloane, "Physician-Patient Communication in the Primary Care Office: A Systematic Review," *Journal of the American Board of Family Practice* 15, no. 1 (2002): 25–38, https://www.jabfm.org/content/jabfp/15/1/25.full.pdf.

13. Ashlinder Gill et al., "'Where Do We Go from Here?' Health System Frustrations Expressed by Patients with Multimorbidity, Their Caregivers and Family Physicians," *Healthcare Policy* 9, no. 4 (2014): 73–89, https://www.longwoods.com/content/23811.

14. Ibid.

15. Phillip B. Miller, Louis J. Goodman, and Timothy B. Norbeck, *In Their Own Words: 12,000 Physicians Reveal Their Thoughts on Medical Practice in America* (New York: Morgan James Publishing, 2010).

16. Dike Drummond, "Physician Burnout: Its Origin, Symptoms, and Five Main Causes," *Family Practice Management* 22, no. 5 (2015): 42–47, https://www.aafp.org/fpm/2015/0900/p42.html.

17. Drummond, "Physician Burnout."

18. Maggie Oman Shannon, ed., *Prayers for Healing: 365 Blessings, Poems, and Meditations from around the World*, intro. Dalai Lama (Berkeley: Conari Press, 2000).

19. Beck, Daughtridge, and Sloane, "Physician-Patient Communication."

20. Tait D. Shanafelt, "Enhancing Meaning in Work: A Prescription for Preventing Physician Burnout and Promoting Patient-Centered Care," *JAMA* 302, no. 12 (2009): 1338–40; Robin A. J. Youngson, *Time to Care: How to Love Your Patients and Your Job* (Seattle: CreateSpace, 2012).

21. Antoine de Saint-Exupéry, *Le Petit Prince* ([Paris]: Gallimard, 1943), first translated into English by Katherine Woods as *The Little Prince* ([New York]: Reynal and Hitchcock, 1943).

Bibliography

Ackoff, Russell Lincoln. *Redesigning the Future: A Systems Approach to Societal Problems.* New York: John Wiley and Sons, 1974.

Advisory Board. "Behind Bars: The Downfall of the Nation's Busiest Cardiologist." October 31, 2013. https://www.advisory.com/Daily-Briefing/2013/10/31/Behind -bars-The-downfall-of-the-nation-busiest-cardiologist.

Aldweib, Nael, Kazuaki Negishi, Rory Hachamovitch, Wael Abdel Jaber, Sinziana Seicean, and Thomas H. Marwick. "Impact of Repeat Myocardial Revascularization on Outcome in Patients with Silent Ischemia after Previous Revascularization." *Journal of the American College of Cardiology* 61, no. 15 (2013): 1616–23. http://www .onlinejacc.org/content/61/15/1616.

Al-Khatib, Sana M., Anne S. Hellkamp, Jeptha S. Curtis, Daniel B. Mark, Eric D. Peterson, Gillian D. Sanders, Paul A. Heidenreich, Adrian F. Hernandez, Lesley H. Curtis, and Stephen C. Hammill. "Non-Evidence-Based ICD Implantations in the United States." *JAMA* 305, no. 1 (2011): 43–49. https://jamanetwork.com/journals/ jama/fullarticle/644551.

American Board of Internal Medicine Foundation. "American College of Cardiology: Five Things Physicians and Patients Should Question." Choosing Wisely (website). Updated February 28, 2017. http://www.choosingwisely.org/societies/american -college-of-cardiology/.

American Heart Association. "Ablation for Arrhythmias." Heart.org. Last reviewed September 30, 2016. https://www.heart.org/en/health-topics/arrhythmia/prevention —treatment-of-arrhythmia/ablation-for-arrhythmias.

———. "Implantable Cardioverter Defibrillator (ICD)." Heart.org. Last reviewed September 30, 2016. http://www.heart.org/en/health-topics/arrhythmia/prevention —treatment-of-arrhythmia/implantable-cardioverter-defibrillator-icd.

————. "Lifestyle Changes for Heart Attack Prevention." Heart.org. Last reviewed July 31, 2015. http://www.heart.org/HEARTORG/Conditions/HeartAttack/LifeAfter aHeartAttack/Lifestyle-Changes-for-Heart-Attack-Prevention_UCM_303934 _Article.jsp.

————. "Tachycardia: Fast Heart Rate." Heart.org. Last reviewed September 30, 2016. http://www.heart.org/en/health-topics/arrhythmia/about-arrhythmia/tachycardia —fast-heart-rate.

————. "What Is Arrhythmia?" 2015. https://www.heart.org/-/media/data-import/ downloadables/pe-abh-what-is-arrhythmia-ucm_300290.pdf.

Anselmino, Matteo, Fabrizio D'Ascenzo, Gisella Amoroso, Frederico Ferraris, and Fiorenzo Gaita. "History of Transcatheter Atrial Fibrillation Ablation." *Journal of Cardiovascular Medicine* 13, no. 1 (2012): 1–8.

Antiarrhythmics Versus Implantable Defibrillators (AVID) Investigators. "A Comparison of Antiarrhythmic-Drug Therapy with Implantable Defibrillators in Patients Resuscitated from Near-Fatal Ventricular Arrhythmias." *The New England Journal of Medicine* 337, no. 22 (1997): 1576–83. https://www.nejm.org/doi/10.1056/ NEJM199711273372202.

Aquilina, O. "A Brief History of Cardiac Pacing." *Images in Paediatric Cardiology* 8, no. 2 (2006): 17–81. https://www.ncbi.nlm.nih.gov/pmc/articles/PMC3232561/.

Bardy, Gust H., Kerry L. Lee, Daniel B. Mark, Jeanne E. Poole, Douglas L. Packer, Robin Boineau, Michael Domanski, et al., for the Sudden Cardiac Death in Heart Failure Trial (SCD-HeFT) Investigators. "Amiodarone or an Implantable Cardioverter-Defibrillator for Congestive Heart Failure." *The New England Journal of Medicine* 352, no. 3 (2005): 225–37. https://www.nejm.org/doi/full/10.1056/ nejmoa043399.

Bar-Eli, Michael, Ofer H. Azar, Ilana Ritov, Yael Keidar-Levin, and Galit Schein. "Action Bias among Elite Soccer Goalkeepers: The Case of Penalty Kicks." *Journal of Economic Psychology* 28, no. 5 (2007): 606–21.

Barger-Lux, M. J., and R. P. Heaney. "For Better and Worse: The Technological Imperative in Health Care." *Social Science and Medicine* 22, no. 12 (1986): 1313–20.

Barnafeder. "Wilson Greatbatch, Inventor of Implantable Pacemaker, Dies at 92." *New York Times*, September 28, 2011. https://www.nytimes.com/2011/09/28/business/ wilson-greatbatch-pacemaker-inventor-dies-at-92.html.

Barra Sérgio, Rui Providência, Luís Paiva, Patrick Heck, and Sharad Agarwal. "Implantable Cardioverter-Defibrillators in the Elderly: Rationale and Specific Age-Related Considerations." *EP Europace* 17, no. 2 (2015): 174–86. https://doi.org/10.1093/ europace/euu296.

Barton, Matthias, Johannes Grüntzig, Marc Husmann, and Josef Rösch. "Balloon Angioplasty—The Legacy of Andreas Grüntzig, M.D. (1939–1985)." *Frontiers in Cardiovascular Medicine* 1, no.15 (2014). http://doi.org/10.3389/fcvm.2014.00015.

Beck, Rainer S., Rebecca Daughtridge, and Philip D. Sloane. "Physician-Patient Communication in the Primary Care Office: A Systematic Review." *Journal of the American Board of Family Practice* 15, no. 1 (2002): 25–38. https://www.jabfm.org/ content/jabfp/15/1/25.full.pdf.

Beller, George A. "Tests that May Be Overused or Misused in Cardiology: The Choosing Wisely Campaign." *Journal of Nuclear Cardiology* 19, no.3 (2012): 401–403. https://link.springer.com/article/10.1007%2Fs12350-012-9569-y.

Ben-Haim, Shlomo. "How Innovation Can Unleash Tremendous Growth in the $3.4 Billion AF Ablation Market." *Cardiac Rhythm News*. February 29, 216. https://cardiacrhythmnews.com/how-innovation-can-unleash-tremendous-growth-in-the-3-4-billion-af-ablation-market/.

Benjamin, Emelia J., Philip A. Wolf, Ralph B. D'Agostino, Halit Silbershatz, William Bernard Kannel, and Daniel Lévy. "Impact of Atrial Fibrillation on the Risk of Death: The Framingham Heart Study." *Circulation* 98, no. 10 (1998): 946–52.

Bennekers, J. H., Rob van Mechelen, and A. Meijer. "Pacemaker Safety and Long-Distance Running." *Netherlands Heart Journal* 12, no. 10 (2004): 450–54. https://www.ncbi.nlm.nih.gov/pmc/articles/PMC2497157/pdf/Nheartj00109-0018.pdf.

Bernstein, Steven J., Marianne Laouri, Lee H. Hilborne, Lucian L. Leape, James P. Kahan, Rolla Edward Park, Caren Kamberg, and Robert H. Brook. "Coronary Angiography: A Literature Review and Ratings of Appropriateness and Necessity." Santa Monica, CA: RAND Corporation, 1992. Available for download at https://www.rand.org/pubs/joint_reports-health/JRA03.html.

Betts, Timothy R., Praveen P. Sadarmin, David R. Tomlinson, Kim Rajappan, Kelvin C. K. Wong, Joseph P. de Bono, and Yaver Bashir. "Absolute Risk Reduction in Total Mortality with Implantable Cardioverter Defibrillators: Analysis of Primary and Secondary Prevention Trial Data to Aid Risk/Benefit Analysis." *EP Europace* 15, no. 6 (2013): 813–19. https://doi.org/10.1093/europace/eus427.

Bilton, Nick. "For Fitness Bands, Slick Marketing but Suspect Results." Bits. *New York Times*, April 27, 2014. https://bits.blogs.nytimes.com/2014/04/27/for-fitness-bands-slick-marketing-but-suspect-results/.

Bishop, Tricia. "Federal Report on Stent Procedures Finds Potential Fraud." *Baltimore Sun*, December 6, 2010. http://articles.baltimoresun.com/2010-12-06/health/bs-md-senate-stent-report-20101205_1_stent-procedures-midei-abbott-brand.

———. "Mark Midei Fights for Medical License, Exoneration." *Baltimore Sun*, December 10, 2011. http://www.baltimoresun.com/health/bs-md-mark-midei-exclusive-20111210-story.html.

Blackburn, Henry. "Donald Reid, MD." University of Minnesota (website). Last modified October 15, 2012. http://www.epi.umn.edu/cvdepi/bio-sketch/reid-donald/.

Boden, William E., Robert A. O'Rourke, Koon K. Teo, Pamela M. Hartigan, David J. Maron, William J. Kostuk, Merril Knudtson, et al. "Optimal Medical Therapy with or without PCI for Stable Coronary Disease." *The New England Journal of Medicine* 356, no. 15 (2007): 1503–16. https://www.nejm.org/doi/full/10.1056/NEJMoa070829.

Böhm, Ádám, Ferenc Bányai, István Préda, and Károly Zámolyi. "The Treatment of Septicemia in Pacemaker Patients." *Pacing and Clinical Electrophysiology* 19, no. 7 (1996): 1105–11.

Borden, William B., Rita F. Redberg, Alvin I. Mushlin, David Dai, Lisa A. Kaltenbach, and John A. Spertus. "Patterns and Intensity of Medical Therapy in Patients

Undergoing Percutaneous Coronary Intervention." *JAMA* 305, no. 18 (2011): 1882–89. https://jamanetwork.com/journals/jama/fullarticle/899881.

Borren, Nanette M., Jan Paul Ottervanger, Martijn A. Reinders, and Elvin Kedhi. "Coronary Artery Stenoses More Often Overestimated in Older Patients: Angiographic Stenosis Overestimation in Elderly." *International Journal of Cardiology* 241 (2017): 46–49.

Bourque, Jamieson M., George T. Charlton, Benjamin H. Holland, Christopher M. Belyea, Denny D. Watson, and George A. Beller. "Prognosis in Patients Achieving ≥ 10 METS on Exercise Stress Testing: Was SPECT Imaging Useful?" *Journal of Nuclear Cardiology* 18, no. 2 (2011): 230–37. https://www.ncbi.nlm.nih.gov/pmc/articles/PMC3902109/.

Bousfield, Guy. "Angina Pectoris: Changes in Electrocardiogram during Paroxysm." *The Lancet* 192, no. 4962 (1918): 457–58.

Bradley, Steven M., John A. Spertus, Kevin F. Kennedy, Brahmajee K. Nallamothu, Paul S. Chan, Manesh R. Patel, Chris L. Bryson, David J. Malenka, and John S. Rumsfield. "Patient Selection for Diagnostic Coronary Angiography and Hospital-Level Percutaneous Coronary Intervention Appropriateness: Insights from the National Cardiovascular Data Registry." *JAMA Internal Medicine* 174, no. 10 (2014): 1630–39. https://jamanetwork.com/journals/jamainternalmedicine/fullarticle/1898877.

Braunwald, Eugene. "Coronary Artery Bypass Surgery—An Assessment." *Postgraduate Medical Journal* 52, no. 614 (1976): 733–38. https://pmj.bmj.com/content/post gradmedj/52/614/733.full.pdf.

Brown, David L., and Rita F. Redberg. "Continuing Use of Prophylactic Percutaneous Coronary Intervention in Patients with Stable Coronary Artery Disease Despite Evidence of No Benefit: Déjà Vu All Over Again." *JAMA Internal Medicine* 176, no. 5 (2016): 597–98.

———. "Last Nail in the Coffin for PCI in Stable Angina?" *The Lancet* 391, no. 10115 (2018): 3–4.

Bruce, R. A., J. R. Blackmon, J. W. Jones, and G. Strait. "Exercise Testing in Adult Normal Subjects and Cardiac Patients." *Pediatrics* 32, no. 4 (1963): 742–56.

Brushchke, Albert V. G., William C. Sheldon, Earl K. Shirey, and William L Proud-fit. "A Half Century of Selective Coronary Arteriography." *Journal of the American College of Cardiology* 54, no. 23 (2009): 2139–44. https://www.sciencedirect.com/science/article/pii/S0735109709030083?via%3Dihub.

Bush, David E., and Thomas E. Finucane. "Permanent Cardiac Pacemakers in the Elderly." *Journal of the American Geriatric Society* 42, no. 3 (1994): 326–34.

Butler, Katy. "What Broke My Father's Heart." *New York Times Magazine*, June 18, 2010. https://www.nytimes.com/2010/06/20/magazine/20pacemaker-t.html.

Buxton, Alfred E., Kerry L. Lee, John D. Fisher, Mark E. Josephson, Eric N. Prystowsky, and Gail E. Hafley. "A Randomized Study of the Prevention of Sudden Death in Patients with Coronary Artery Disease. Multicenter Unsustained Tachycardia Trial Investigators." *The New England Journal of Medicine* 341, no. 25 (1999): 1882–90. https://www.nejm.org/doi/10.1056/NEJM199912163412503.

Byrd, Charles L., Bruce L. Wilkoff, Charles J. Love, T. Duncan Sellers, Kyong T. Turk, Russell C. Reeves, Rob J. Young, et al. "Intravascular Extraction of Problematic or Infected Permanent Pacemaker Leads: 1994–1996. U.S. Extraction Database, MED Institute." *Pacing and Clinical Electrophysiology* 22, no. 9 (1999): 1348–57.

Cadmus-Bertram, Lisa, Ronald Gangnon, Emily J. Wirkus, Keith M. Thraen-Borowski, and Jessica Gorzelitz-Liebhauser. "The Accuracy of Heart Rate Monitoring by Some Wrist-Worn Activity Trackers." *Annals of Internal Medicine* 166, no. 8 (2017): 610–12.

Caldeira, Daniel, Cláudio David, and Cristina Sampaio. "Rate vs Rhythm Control in Patients with Atrial Fibrillation and Heart Failure: A Systematic Review and Meta-Analysis of Randomised Controlled Trials." *European Journal of Internal Medicine* 22, no. 5 (2011): 448–55.

Camm, A. John, Günter Breithardt, Harry J. G. M. Crijns, Paul Dorian, Peter Russell Kowey, Jean-Yves Le Heuzey, Ihsen Merioua, Laurence Pedrazzini, Eric N. Prystowsky, Peter J. Schwartz, Christian Torp-Pedersen, and William Weintraub. "Real-Life Observations of Clinical Outcomes with Rhythm- and Rate-Control Therapies for Atrial Fibrillation: RECORDAF (Registry on Cardiac Rhythm Disorders Assessing the Control of Atrial Fibrillation)." *Journal of the American College of Cardiology* 58, no. 5 (2011): 493–501. http://www.onlinejacc.org/content/58/5/493.full.

CBS News, Associated Press. "15-Minute-Old Premature Newborn Receives Pacemaker." Updated February 16, 2012. https://www.cbsnews.com/news/15-minute-old-premature-newborn-receives-pacemaker/.

Centers for Disease Control and Prevention. "Atrial Fibrillation Fact Sheet." CDC. gov. Last reviewed August 22, 2017. https://www.cdc.gov/dhdsp/data_statistics/fact_sheets/fs_atrial_fibrillation.htm.

Chan, Paul S., Sunil V. Rao, Deepak L. Bhatt, John S. Rumsfeld, Hitinder S. Gurm, Brahmajee K. Nallamothu, Matthew A. Cavender, Kevin F. Kennedy, and John A. Spertus. "Patient and Hospital Characteristics Associated with Inappropriate Percutaneous Coronary Interventions." *Journal of the American College of Cardiology* 62, no. 24 (2013): 2274–81. https://doi.org/10.1016/j.jacc.2013.07.086.

Chan, Sue. "Surgery for Profit?" CBS News. November 21, 2002. https://www.cbsnews.com/news/surgery-for-profit/.

Chang, Andrew Y., Daniel W. Kaiser, Aditya Jathin Ullal, Alexander Carroll Perino, Paul A. Heidenreich, and Mintu P. Turakhia. "Evaluating the Cost-Effectiveness of Catheter Ablation of Atrial Fibrillation." *Arrhythmia and Electrophysiology Review* 3, no. 3 (2014): 177–83. https://www.ncbi.nlm.nih.gov/pmc/articles/PMC4711535/.

Ching, Chor Kwan, Ying Hoo Lam, Albert Y. W. Chan, and Tony W. L. Mak. "Adulteration of Herbal Antidiabetic Products with Undeclared Pharmaceuticals: A Case Series in Hong Kong." *British Journal of Clinical Pharmacology* 73, no. 5 (2012): 795–800. https://doi.org/10.1111/j.1365-2125.2011.04135.x.

Cohen, Rebecca J., Kirsten Ek, and Cynthia X. Pan. "Complementary and Alternative Medicine (CAM) Use by Older Adults: A Comparison of Self-Report and Physician Chart Documentation." *The Journals of Gerontology: Series A* 57, no. 4 (2002): M223–27. https://doi.org/10.1093/gerona/57.4.M223.

Croskerry, Pat. "The Importance of Cognitive Errors in Diagnosis and Strategies to Minimize Them." *Academic Medicine* 78, no. 8 (2003): 775–80. https://journals .lww.com/academicmedicine/Fulltext/2003/08000/The_Importance_of_Cognitive _Errors_in_Diagnosis.3.aspx.

Dalcher, Darren. *Further Advances in Project Management: Guided Exploration in Unfamiliar Landscapes*. London: Routledge, 2016.

Dartmouth Atlas Project. *Cardiac Surgery Report*. Dartmouth Atlas of Health Care: Studies of Surgical Variation, 2005. Center for the Evaluative Clinical Sciences. http://archive.dartmouthatlas.org/downloads/reports/Cardiac_report_2005.pdf.

———. "General FAQ." Visited January 23, 2018. https://www.dartmouthatlas.org/faq/.

Desai, Nihar R., Steven M. Bradley, Craig S. Parzynski, Brahmajee K. Nallamothu, Paul S. Chan, John A. Spertus, Manesh R. Patel, Jeremy Ader, Aaron Soufer, Harlan M. Krumholz, and Jeptha P. Curtis. "Appropriate Use Criteria for Coronary Revascularization and Trends in Utilization, Patient Selection, and Appropriateness of Percutaneous Coronary Intervention." *JAMA* 314, no. 19 (2015): 2045–53. https:// jamanetwork.com/journals/jama/fullarticle/2469192.

Deshmukh, Abhishek, Nileshkumar Jasmatbhai Patel, Sadip Pant, Neeraj Shah, Ankit Chothani, Kathan Mehta, Peeyush M. Grover, et al. "In-Hospital Complications Associated with Catheter Ablation of Atrial Fibrillation in the United States between 2000 and 2010: Analysis of 93 801 Procedures." *Circulation* 128, no. 19 (2013): 2104–12. https://doi.org/10.1161/CIRCULATIONAHA.113.003862.

Deyell, Marc W., Stanley Tung, and Adrew Ignaszewski. "The Implantable Cardioverter-Defibrillator: From Mirowski to Its Current Use." *BC Medical Journal* 52, no. 5 (2010): 248–53. https://www.bcmj.org/articles/implantable-cardioverter -defibrillator-mirowski-its-current-use.

Doris, Edward, Iain Matthews, and Honey Thomas. "Heart Rate Monitors and Fitness Trackers: Friend or Foe?" *British Journal of Cardiology* 24 (2017): 137–41.

Drummond, Dike. "Physician Burnout: Its Origin, Symptoms, and Five Main Causes." *Family Practice Management* 22, no. 5 (2015): 42–47. https://www.aafp .org/fpm/2015/0900/p42.html.

Dwyer-Lindgren, Laura, Amelia Bertozzi-Villa, Rebecca W. Stubbs, Chloe Morozoff, Johan Pieter Mackenbach, Frank J. van Lenthe, Ali H. Mokdad, and Christopher J. L. Murray. "Inequalities in Life Expectancy among US Counties, 1980 to 2014: Temporal Trends and Key Drivers." *JAMA Internal Medicine* 177, no. 7 (2017): 1003–11. https://jamanetwork.com/journals/jamainternalmedicine/fullarticle/ 2626194.

Eichenwald, Kurt. "Operating Profits: Mining Medicare; How One Hospital Benefited from Questionable Surgery." *New York Times*, August 12, 2003. https://www .nytimes.com/2003/08/12/business/operating-profits-mining-medicare-one-hospital -benefited-questionable-surgery.html.

Eisenberg, David M., Roger B. Davis, Susan L. Ettner, Scott Appel, Sonja Wilkey, Maria Van Rompay, and Ronald C. Kessler. "Trends in Alternative Medicine Use in the United States, 1990–1997: Results of a Follow-Up National Survey." *JAMA* 280, no. 18 (1998): 1569–75. https://jamanetwork.com/journals/jama/fullarticle/188148.

Eisler, Peter, and Barbara Hansen. "Doctors Perform Thousands of Unnecessary Surgeries." *USA Today*. Updated June 20, 2013. https://www.usatoday.com/story/news/nation/2013/06/18/unnecessary-surgery-usa-today-investigation/2435009/.

Emanuel, Ezekiel J. "Are Good Doctors Bad for Your Health?" *New York Times*, November 21, 2015. https://www.nytimes.com/2015/11/22/opinion/sunday/are-good-doctors-bad-for-your-health.html.

Encyclopedia.com. S.v. "Hales, Stephen." Accessed July 3, 2018. https://www.encyclopedia.com/people/science-and-technology/biology-biographies/stephen-hales.

Epstein, Andrew J., Daniel Polsky, Feifei Yang, Lin Yang, and Peter W. Groeneveld. "Coronary Revascularization Trends in the United States, 2001–2008." *JAMA* 305, no. 17 (2011): 1769–76. https://jamanetwork.com/journals/jama/fullarticle/899648.

Ernst, E. "Adulteration of Chinese Herbal Medicines with Synthetic Drugs: A Systematic Review." *Journal of Internal Medicine* 252, no. 2 (2002): 107–13. https://doi.org/10.1046/j.1365-2796.2002.00999.x.

Evans, Jonathan St. B. T., Stephen E. Newstead, and Ruth M. J. Byrne. *Human Reasoning: The Psychology of Deduction*. Hillsdale, NJ: Lawrence Erlbaum Associates, 1993.

Fairfield, Kathleen M., Adam W. Black, F. Lee Lucas, Andrea E. Siewers, Mylan C. Cohen, Christopher T. Healey, Allison C. Briggs, Paul K. J. Han, and John E. Wennberg. "Behavioral Risk Factors and Regional Variation in Cardiovascular Health Care and Death." *American Journal of Preventive Medicine* 54, no. 3 (2018): 376–84.

Fetters, K. Aleisha. "6 Myths about Nutritional Supplements You Must Know." *U.S. News and World Report*, April 27, 2018. https://health.usnews.com/wellness/food/articles/2018-04-27/6-myths-about-nutritional-supplements-you-must-know.

Fihn, Stephan D., Julius M. Gardin, Jonathan Abrams, Kathleen Berra, James C. Blankenship, Apostolos P. Dallas, Pamela Sylvia Douglas, et al. "2012 ACCF / AHA / ACP / AATS / PCNA / SCAI / STS Guideline for the Diagnosis and Management of Patients with Stable Ischemic Heart Disease: Executive Summary." *Circulation* 126, no. 25 (2012): 3097–3137. https://www.ahajournals.org/doi/10.1161/CIR.0b013e3182776f83.

Fisher, Elliott S., David E. Wennberg, Thérèse A. Stukel, Daniel J. Gottlieb, Frances Leslie Lucas, and Étoile L. Pinder. "The Implications of Regional Variations in Medicare Spending. Part 1: The Content, Quality, and Accessibility of Care." *Annals of Internal Medicine* 138, no. 4 (2003): 273–87. http://annals.org/aim/fullarticle/716066/implications-regional-variations-medicare-spending-part-1-content-quality-accessibility.

Fleisher, Lee A., Kirsten E. Fleischmann, Andrew D. Auerbach, Susan A. Barnason, Joshua A. Beckman, Biykem Bozkurt, Victor G. Davila-Roman, et al. "2014 ACC/AHA Guideline on Perioperative Cardiovascular Evaluation and Management of Patients Undergoing Noncardiac Surgery: A Report of the American College of Cardiology/American Heart Association Task Force on Practice Guidelines." *Journal of the American College of Cardiology* 64, no. 22 (2014): e77–137. http://www.onlinejacc.org/content/64/22/e77.

Freeman, David. "The Truth about Heart Rate and Exercise." WebMD, October 23, 2009. https://www.webmd.com/fitness-exercise/features/the-truth-about-heart-rate-and-exercise#1.

Fukunishi, Masanori, Kazuhiko Nishigaki, Munenori Okubo, Masanori Kawasaki, Genzou Takemura, Shinya Minatoguchi, and Hisayoshi Fujiwara. "J-SAP Study 1–2: Outcomes of Patients with Stable High-Risk Coronary Artery Disease Receiving Medical-Preceding Therapy in Japan." *Circulation* 70, no. 8 (2006): 1012–16.

Fuster, Valentin, Lars E. Rydén, Davis S. Cannom, Harry J. Crijns, Anne B. Curtis, Kenneth A. Ellenbogen, Jonathan L. Halperin, et al. "2011 ACCF/AHA/HRS Focused Updates Incorporated into the ACC/AHA/ESC 2006 Guidelines for the Management of Patients with Atrial Fibrillation: A Report of the American College of Cardiology Foundation/American Heart Association Task Force on Practice Guidelines." *Circulation* 123, no. 10 (2011): e269–367. https://doi.org/10.1161/CIR.0b013e318214876d.

Fye, W. Bruce. "A History of the Origin, Evolution, and Impact of Electrocardiography." *American Journal of Cardiology* 73, no. 13 (1994): 937–49.

Ganz, Leonard I. "Overview of Catheter Ablation of Cardiac Arrhythmias." *UpToDate*, Wolters Kluwer. Last updated January 24, 2019. https://www.uptodate.com/contents/overview-of-catheter-ablation-of-cardiac-arrhythmias (subscription required).

Geller, Andrew I., Nadine Shehab, Nina J. Weidle, Maribeth C. Lovegrove, Beverly J. Wolpert, Babgaleh B. Timbo, Robert P. Mozersky, and Daniel S. Budnitz. "Emergency Department Visits for Adverse Events Related to Dietary Supplements." *The New England Journal of Medicine* 373, no. 16 (2015): 1531–40. https://www.nejm.org/doi/full/10.1056/nejmsa1504267.

Gerber, Yariv, Charanjit S. Rihal, Thoralf M. Sundt, Jill M. Killian, Susan A. Weston, Terry M. Therneau, and Véronique L. Roger. "Coronary Revascularization in the Community: A Population-Based Study, 1990 to 2004." *Journal of the American College of Cardiology* 50, no. 13 (2007): 1223–29. https://doi.org/10.1016/j.jacc.2007.06.022.

Gill, Ashlinder, Kerry Kuluski, Liisa Jaakkimainen, Gayathri Naganathan, Ross E. G. Upshur, and Walter P. Wodchis. "'Where Do We Go from Here?' Health System Frustrations Expressed by Patients with Multimorbidity, Their Caregivers and Family Physicians." *Healthcare Policy* 9, no. 4 (2014): 73–89. https://www.longwoods.com/content/23811.

Gillum, Richard F. "Coronary Artery Bypass Surgery and Coronary Angiography in the United States, 1979–1983." *American Heart Journal* 113, no. 5 (1987): 1255–60.

Glamour. "Why You Should Never Google Your Symptoms." Well + Good. September 25, 2015. https://www.glamour.com/story/why-you-should-never-google-yo.

Goff, Sarah L., Kathleen M. Mazor, Henry H. Ting, Reva W. Kleppel, and Michael B. Rothberg. "How Cardiologists Present the Benefits of Percutaneous Coronary Interventions to Patients with Stable Angina: A Qualitative Analysis." *JAMA Internal Medicine* 174, no. 10 (2014): 1614–21. https://jamanetwork.com/journals/jamainternalmedicine/fullarticle/1898875.

Gonzalez, Rolando, Melvin Scheinman, William Margaretten, and Michael Rubinstein. "Closed-Chest Electrode-Catheter Technique for His Bundle Ablation in Dogs." *American Journal of Physiology* 241, no. 2 (1981): H283–87.

Goodney, Philip P., Karina A. Newhall, Kimon Bekelis, Daniel Gottlieb, Richard Comi, Sushela Chaudrain, Adrienne E. Faerber, Todd A. Mackenzie, and Jonathan

S. Skinner. "Consistency of Hemoglobin A1c Testing and Cardiovascular Outcomes in Medicare Patients with Diabetes." *Journal of the American Heart Association* 5, no. 8 (2016): e003566. https://www.ncbi.nlm.nih.gov/pmc/articles/PMC5015285/.

Greenberg, A., P. R. Kowey, E. Bargmann, and S. M. Wolfe. "Permanent Pacemakers in Maryland." Report. Washington, DC: Health Research Group, 1982.

Greenspan, Allan M., Harold R. Kay, Bruce C. Berger, Richard M. Greenberg, Arnold J. Greenspon, and Mary Jane Spuhler Gaughan. "Incidence of Unwarranted Implantation of Permanent Cardiac Pacemakers in a Large Medical Population." *The New England Journal of Medicine* 318, no. 3 (1988): 158–63.

Groopman, Jerome. *How Doctors Think*. Boston: Mariner Books, 2008.

Gross, Annette S., Yan D. Goh, Russell S. Addison, and Gillian M. Shenfield. "Influence of Grapefruit Juice on Cisapride Pharmacokinetics." *Clinical Pharmacology and Therapeutics* 65, no. 4 (1999): 395–401.

Haegli, Laurent M., and Hugh Calkins. "Catheter Ablation of Atrial Fibrillation: An Update." *European Heart Journal* 35, no. 36 (2014): 2454–59. https://doi.org/10.1093/eurheartj/ehu291.

Haïssaguerre, Michel, Pierre Jaïs, Dipen Chandrakant Shah, Atsushi Takahashi, Mélèze Hocini, Gilles Quiniou, Stéphane X. Garrigue, Alain Le Mouroux, Philippe Le Métayer, and Jacques Clémenty. "Spontaneous Initiation of Atrial Fibrillation by Ectopic Beats Originating in the Pulmonary Veins." *The New England Journal of Medicine* 339, no. 10 (1998): 659–66. https://www.nejm.org/doi/full/10.1056/NEJM199809033391003.

Hannan, Edward L., Kimberly S. Cozzens, Zaza Samadashvili, Gary Walford, Alice K. Jacobs, David R. Holmes Jr., Nicholas J. Stamato, Samin K. Sharma, Ferdinand J. Venditti, Icilma V. Fergus, and Spencer B. King III. "Appropriateness of Coronary Revascularization for Patients without Acute Coronary Syndromes." *Journal of the American College of Cardiology* 59, no. 21 (2012): 1870–76. http://www.onlinejacc.org/content/59/21/1870.

Hannan, Edward L., Zaza Samadashvili, Kimberly Cozzens, Gary Walford, David R. Holmes Jr., Alice K. Jacobs, Nicholas J. Stamato, Ferdinand J. Venditti, Samin Sharma, and Spencer B. King III. "Appropriateness of Diagnostic Catheterization for Suspected Coronary Artery Disease in New York State." *Circulation: Cardiovascular Interventions* 7, no. 1 (2014): 19–27. https://www.ahajournals.org/doi/10.1161/CIRCINTERVENTIONS.113.000741.

Harb, Serge C., Thomas Cook, Wael A. Jaber, and Thomas H. Marwick. "Exercise Testing in Asymptomatic Patients after Revascularization: Are Outcomes Altered?" *Archives of Internal Medicine* 172, no.11 (2012): 854–61. https://jamanetwork.com/journals/jamainternalmedicine/fullarticle/1151706.

Hart, Robert G., Oscar R. Benavente, Rocky McBride, and Lesly A. Pearce. "Antithrombotic Therapy to Prevent Stroke in Patients with Atrial Fibrillation: A Meta-Analysis." *Annals of Internal Medicine* 131, no. 7 (1999): 492–501. http://annals.org/aim/fullarticle/712970/therapy-prevent-stroke-patients-atrial-fibrillation.

Harvard Health Publishing. "Shocking News: Overdoing ICDs." *Harvard Health Letter*. March 2011. https://www.health.harvard.edu/heart-health/shocking-news-overdoing-icds (subscription required).

Harvard Men's Health Watch. "Cardiac Exercise Stress Testing: What It Can and Cannot Tell You." Harvard Health Publishing. Updated August 22, 2018. https:// www.health.harvard.edu/heart-disease-overview/cardiac-exercise-stress-testing-what -it-can-and-cannot-tell-you.

Head, Stuart J., Teresa M. Kieser, Volkmar Falk, Hans A. Huysmans, and A. Pieter Kappetein. "Coronary Artery Bypass Grafting: Part 1—The Evolution Over the First 50 Years." *European Heart Journal* 34, no. 37 (2013): 2862–72. https://doi .org/10.1093/eurheartj/eht330.

Hefflin, Brockton J. "Final-Year-of-Life Pacemaker Recipients." *Journal of the American Geriatrics Society* 46, no.11 (1998): 1396–400.

Helm, Janet. "Getting to the Root of the Turmeric Trend." *Nutrition Unplugged.* June 6, 2015. https://www.nutritionunplugged.com/2015/06/getting-root-turmeric-trend/.

Hexa Research. "Herbal Medicine Market Size and Forecast, by Product (Tablets and Capsules, Powders, Extracts), by Indication (Digestive Disorders, Respiratory Disorders, Blood Disorders), and Trend Analysis, 2014–2024." September 2017. https:// www.hexaresearch.com/research-report/global-herbal-medicine-market.

Hillis, L. David, Peter K. Smith, Jeffrey L. Anderson, John A. Bittl, Charles R. Bridges, John G. Byrne, Joaquin E. Cigarroa, et al. "2011 ACCF/AHA Guideline for Coronary Artery Bypass Graft Surgery: A Report of the American College of Cardiology Foundation/American Heart Association Task Force on Practice Guidelines." *Circulation* 124, no. 23 (2011): e652–e735. https://doi.org/10.1161/ CIR.0b013e31823c074e.

Huang, Xiaoyan, and Meredith B. Rosenthal. "Overuse of Cardiovascular Services: Evidence, Causes, and Opportunities for Reform." *Circulation* 132, no. 3 (2015): 205–14. https://www.ahajournals.org/doi/full/10.1161/CIRCULATION AHA.114.012668.

Husten, Larry. "Mark Midei Can't Get a Job Taking Blood Pressure at a Walmart." *Forbes,* April 8, 2012. https://www.forbes.com/sites/larryhusten/2012/04/08/mark -midei-cant-get-a-job-taking-blood-pressure-at-a-walmart/.

January, Craig, T., L. Samuel Wann, Joseph S. Alpert, Hugh Calkins, Joaquin E. Cigarroa, Joseph C. Cleveland Jr., Jamie B. Conti, et al. "2014 AHA/ACC/HRS Guideline for the Management of Patients with Atrial Fibrillation: Executive Summary." *Journal of the American College of Cardiology* 64, no. 21 (2014): 2246–80. http:// www.onlinejacc.org/content/64/21/2246.

Jefferies, John Lynn, and Jeffrey A. Towbin. "Dilated Cardiomyopathy." *The Lancet* 375, no. 9716 (2010): 752–62.

Jefferson, Thomas. *The Works of Thomas Jefferson in Twelve Volumes.* Federal edition. Collected and edited by Paul Leicester Ford. New York, London: G. P. Putnam's Sons, 1904–1905.

Jeffrey, Kirk, and Victor Parsonnet. "Cardiac Pacing, 1960–1985: A Quarter Century of Medical and Industrial Innovation." *Circulation* 97, no. 19 (1998): 1978–91.

Jena, Anupam B., Vinay Prasad, Dana P. Goldman, and John Romley. "Mortality and Treatment Patterns among Patients Hospitalized with Acute Cardiovascular Conditions during Dates of National Cardiology Meetings." *JAMA Internal Medicine* 175, no. 2 (2015): 237–44. https://jamanetwork.com/journals/jamainternalmedicine/fullarticle/2038979.

Joseph, J. P., and K. Rajappan. "Radiofrequency Ablation of Cardiac Arrhythmias: Past, Present and Future." *QJM* 105, no. 4 (2012): 303–14. https://doi.org/10.1093/qjmed/hcr189.

Kahneman, Daniel. *Thinking, Fast and Slow*. New York: Farrar, Straus and Giroux, 2013.

Keller, Benjamin. "Self-Tracking, to the Point of Obsession." *In Vivo*, November 12, 2014. http://www.invivomagazine.com/en/corpore_sano/tendances/article/66/self-tracking-to-the-point-of-obsession.

Kim, Jeongeun, and Sukwha Kim. "Physicians' Perception of the Effects of Internet Health Information on the Doctor–Patient Relationship." *Informatics for Health and Social Care* 34, no. 3 (2009): 136–48.

Kim, Michael H., Stephen S. Johnston, Bong-Chul Chu, Mehul R. Dalal, and Kathy L. Schulman. "Estimation of Total Incremental Health Care Costs in Patients with Atrial Fibrillation in the United States." *Circulation: Cardiovascular Quality Outcomes* 4, no. 3 (2011): 313–20. https://doi.org/10.1161/CIRCOUTCOMES.110.958165.

Kimmel, Stephen E., Jesse A. Berlin, Sean Hennessy, Brian L. Strom, Ronald J. Krone, and Warren K. Laskey for the Registry Committee of the Society for Cardiac Angiography and Interventions. "Risk of Major Complications from Coronary Angioplasty Performed Immediately after Diagnostic Coronary Angiography: Results from the Registry of the Society for Cardiac Angiography and Interventions." *Journal of the American College of Cardiology* 30, no. 1 (1997): 193–200. https://www.sciencedirect.com/science/article/pii/S0735109797001496.

King, Spencer B., III "Angioplasty from Bench to Bedside to Bench." *Circulation* 93, no. 9 (1996): 1621–29. https://www.ahajournals.org/doi/10.1161/01.CIR.93.9.1621.

Kini, Vinay, Elias J. Dayoub, Paul L. Hess, Lucas N. Marzec, Frederick A. Masoudi, P. Michael Ho, and Peter W. Groeneveld. "Clinical Outcomes after Cardiac Stress Testing among US Patients Younger than 65 Years." *Journal of the American Heart Association* 7, no. 6 (2018): e007854. https://www.ahajournals.org/doi/10.1161/JAHA.117.007854.

Klaidman, Stephen. *Coronary: A True Story of Medicine Gone Awry*. New York: Scribner, 2007.

Kolata, Gina. "'Maximum' Heart Rate Theory Is Challenged." *New York Times*, April 24, 2001. https://www.nytimes.com/2001/04/24/health/maximum-heart-rate-theory-is-challenged.html.

Konstantinov, Igor E. "Vasilii I Kolesov: A Surgeon to Remember." *Texas Heart Institute Journal* 31, no. 4 (2004): 349–58. https://www.ncbi.nlm.nih.gov/pmc/articles/PMC548233/.

Kowey, Peter Russell, Allen Greenberg, Eve Bargmann, and Sidney Manuel Wolfe. "State of Maryland Pacemaker Experience (1979–1980): Conflicting Views regarding the Frequency of Unnecessary Pacemaker Implants." *The American Journal of Cardiology* 51, no. 6 (1983): 1042–43.

Krahn, Andrew D., Stuart J. Connolly, Robin S. Roberts, and Michael Gent. "Diminishing Proportional Risk of Sudden Death with Advancing Age: Implications for Prevention of Sudden Death." *American Heart Journal* 147, no. 5 (2004): 837–40.

Kuo, Grace M., Sarah T. Hawley, L. Todd Weiss, Rajesh Balkrishnan, and Robert J. Volk. "Factors Associated with Herbal Use among Urban Multiethnic Primary Care Patients: A Cross-Sectional Survey." *BMC Complementary and Alternative Medicine* 4 (2004): 18. https://doi.org/10.1186/1472-6882-4-18.

Kusumoto, Fred M., Mark H. Schoenfeld, Coletta Barrett, James R. Edgerton, Kenneth A. Ellenbogen, Michael R. Gold, Nora F. Goldschlager, et al. "2018 ACC/AHA/HRS Guideline on the Evaluation and Management of Patients with Bradycardia and Cardiac Conduction Delay." *Journal of the American College of Cardiology* (2018). https://doi.org/10.1016/j.jacc.2018.10.043.

Ladapo, Joseph A., Saul Blecker, and Pamela Sylvia Douglas. "Physician Decision Making and Trends in the Use of Cardiac Stress Testing in the United States: An Analysis of Repeated Cross-Sectional Data." *Annals of Internal Medicine* 161, no. 7 (2014): 482–90.

Leape, Lucian L., Rolla Edward Park, Thomas M. Bashore, John Kevin Harrison, Charles J. Davidson, and Robert H. Brook. "Effect of Variability in the Interpretation of Coronary Angiograms on the Appropriateness of Use of Coronary Revascularization Procedures." *American Heart Journal* 139, no. 1 (2000): 106–13. https://www.sciencedirect.com/science/article/pii/S0002870300700160?via%3Dihub.

Lee, Marion A., Fred Morady, Frank Pelosid Morady, Abraham Kadish, D. J. Schamp, Michael C. Chin, Melvin M. Scheinman, Jerry C. Griffin, Michael D. Lesh, David R. Pederson, and Jacob Goldberger. "Catheter Modification of the Atrioventricular Junction with Radiofrequency Energy for Control of Atrioventricular Nodal Reentry Tachycardia." *Circulation* 83, no. 3 (1991): 827–35.

Levi, Ran. "The Unbelievable Story behind the Invention of Cardiac Catheterization." *Medium* (website). February 17, 2016. https://medium.com/@ranlevi/the-unbelievable-story-behind-the-invention-of-cardiac-catheterization-ac09640cb92d.

Lin, Grace A., R. Adams Dudley, and Rita F. Redberg. "Cardiologists' Use of Percutaneous Coronary Interventions for Stable Coronary Artery Disease." *Archives of Internal Medicine* 167, no. 15 (2007): 1604–1609. https://jamanetwork.com/journals/jamainternalmedicine/fullarticle/769857.

———. "Why Physicians Favor Use of Percutaneous Coronary Intervention to Medical Therapy: A Focus Group Study." *Journal of General Internal Medicine* 23, no. 9 (2008): 1458–63. https://www.ncbi.nlm.nih.gov/pmc/articles/PMC2518034/.

Lip, Gregory Y. H., and D. Gareth Beevers. "ABC of Atrial Fibrillation: History, Epidemiology, and Importance of Atrial Fibrillation." *British Medical Journal* 311, no. 7016 (1995): 1361–63.

Lip, Gregory Y. H., Robby Nieuwlaat, Ron Pisters, Deirdre A. Lane, and Harry J. G. M. Crijns. "Refining Clinical Risk Stratification for Predicting Stroke and Thromboembolism in Atrial Fibrillation Using a Novel Risk Factor-Based Approach: The Euro Heart Survey on Atrial Fibrillation." *Chest* 137, no. 2 (2010): 263–72.

Lown, Bernard, and Paul Axelrod. "Implanted Standby Defibrillators." *Circulation* 46, no. 4 (1972): 637–39. https://www.ahajournals.org/doi/pdf/10.1161/01 .CIR.46.4.637.

Lucas, F. L., Michael A. DeLorenzo, Andrea E. Siewers, and David E. Wennberg. "Temporal Trends in the Utilization of Diagnostic Testing and Treatments for Cardiovascular Disease in the United States, 1993–2001." *Circulation* 113, no. 3 (2006): 374–79. https://www.ahajournals.org/doi/full/10.1161/CIRCULATION AHA.105.560433.

Lüderitz, Berndt. "Historical Perspectives on Interventional Electrophysiology." *Journal of Interventional Cardiac Electrophysiology* 9, no. 2 (2003): 75–83.

Maisel, William H., Michael O. Sweeney, William G. Stevenson, Kristin E. Ellison, and Laurence M. Epstein. "Recalls and Safety Alerts Involving Pacemakers and Implantable Cardioverter-Defibrillator Generators." *JAMA* 286, no.7 (2001): 793–99. https://jamanetwork.com/journals/jama/fullarticle/194108.

Malhotra, Aseem, Rita F. Redberg, and Pascal Meier. "Saturated Fat Does Not Clog the Arteries: Coronary Heart Disease Is a Chronic Inflammatory Condition, the Risk of Which Can Be Effectively Reduced from Healthy Lifestyle Interventions." *British Journal of Sports Medicine* 51, no. 15 (2017): 1111–12. http://dx.doi.org/10.1136/ bjsports-2016-097285.

Mandrola, John. "AF Ablation Is Overused in the US." *Dr. John M* (website). March 11, 2017. http://www.drjohnm.org/2017/03/af-ablation-is-overused-in-the-us/.

Marcus, Gregory M., Derrick W. Chan, and Rita F. Redberg. "Recollection of Pain Due to Inappropriate versus Appropriate Implantable Cardioverter-Defibrillator Shocks." *Pacing and Clinical Electrophysiology* 34, no. 3 (2011): 348–53.

Market Research Future. "Future Trend of Herbal Medicine Market 2018 Scope | at a CAGR of ~7.2% during 2017 to 2023 | Increasing Demand for Safe Therapies." Reuters. April 12 2018. https://www.reuters.com/brandfeatures/venture-capital/ article?id=32992.

Martinelli, Martino, Roberto Costa, Silvana D. Orio Nishioka, Anísio Alexandre Andrade Pedrosa, Sérgio de Freitas Siqueira, Elizabeth Sartori Crevelari, Maurício Scanavacca, André d'Avila, and Eduardo Sosa. "Criteria for Pacemaker Explant in Patients without a Precise Indication for Pacemaker Implantation." *Pacing and Clinical Electrophysiology* 25, no. 3 (2002): 272–77.

Maslow, Abraham H. *The Psychology of Science: A Reconnaissance.* New York: Harper and Row, 1966.

Masoudi, Frederick A., Angelo Ponirakis, James A. de Lemos, James G. Jollis, Mark Kremers, John C. Messenger, John W. M. Moore, et al. "Trends in U.S. Cardiovascular Care: 2016 Report from 4 ACC National Cardiovascular Data Registries." *Journal of the American College of Cardiology* 69, no. 11 (2017): 1427–50. https:// doi.org/10.1016/j.jacc.2016.12.005.

Master, Arthur M., Rudolph Friedman, and Simon Dack. "The Electrocardiogram after Standard Exercise as a Functional Test of the Heart." *American Heart Journal* 24, no. 6 (1942): 777–93.

Matlock, Daniel D., Pamela N. Peterson, Paul A. Heidenreich, F. Lee Lucas, David J. Malenka, Yongfei Wang, Jeptha P. Curtis, Jean Kutner, Elliott Fisher, and Frederick A. Masoudi. "Regional Variation in the Use of Implantable Cardioverter-Defibrillators for Primary Prevention: Results from the National Cardiovascular Data Registry." *Circulation. Cardiovascular Quality and Outcomes* 4, no. 1 (2011): 114–21. https://www.ahajournals.org/doi/10.1161/CIRC OUTCOMES.110.958264.

Mayo Clinic Staff. "Ventricular Tachycardia." Mayo Clinic (website). October 4, 2018. https://www.mayoclinic.org/diseases-conditions/ventricular-tachycardia/symptoms -causes/syc-20355138.

McBride, Sarah. "The Real Me." *The Huffington Post*. May 9, 2012. https://www .huffingtonpost.com/sarah-mcbride/the-real-me_b_1504207.html.

McIntosh, H. D., and J. A. Garcia. "The First Decade of Aortocoronary Bypass Grafting, 1967–1977. A Review." *Circulation* 57, no. 3 (1978): 405–31. https://doi org/10.1161/01.CIR.57.3.405.

McMichael, John. "History of Atrial Fibrillation 1628–1819: Harvey–de Senac–Laënnec." British Heart Journal 48, no. 3 (1982): 193–97. https://www.ncbi.nlm.nih.gov/pmc/ articles/PMC481228/.

Medtronic. *Implantable Cardioverter-Defibrillators (ICDs)*. 2015. https://www .medtronic.com/content/dam/medtronic-com/us-en/newsroom/media-resources/ media-kits/implantable-cardioverter-defibrillators/documents/icd-backgrounder-2015 .pdf.

Miller, D. W., T. D. Ivey, W. W. Bailey, D. D. Johnson, and E. A. Hessel. "The Practice of Coronary Artery Bypass Surgery in 1980." *Journal of Thoracic Cardiovascular Surgery* 81, no. 3 (1981): 423–27.

Miller, Phillip B., Louis J. Goodman, and Timothy B. Norbeck. *In Their Own Words: 12,000 Physicians Reveal Their Thoughts on Medical Practice in America*. New York: Morgan James Publishing, 2010.

Miller, Todd D., Rita F. Redberg, and Frans J. T. Wackers. "Screening Asymptomatic Diabetic Patients for Coronary Artery Disease: Why Not?" *Journal of the American College of Cardiology* 48, no. 4 (2006): 761–64. https://doi.org/10.1016/j .jacc.2006.04.076.

Morady, Fred. "Catheter Ablation of Supraventricular Arrhythmias: State of the Art." *Pacing and Clinical Electrophysiology* 27, no. 1 (2004): 125–42.

Morady, Fred, and Melvin M. [Scheinman]. "Transvenous Catheter Ablation of a Posteroseptal Accessory Pathway in a Patient with the Wolff-Parkinson-White Syndrome." *The New England Journal of Medicine* 310 (1984): 705–707.

Moss, Arthur J., W. Jackson Hall, David S. Cannom, James P. Daubert, Steven L. Higgins, Helmut Klein, Joseph H. Levine, S. Saksena, Albert L. Waldo, David Wilber, Mary W. Brown, and Moonseong Heo. "Improved Survival with an Implanted Defibrillator in Patients with Coronary Disease at High Risk for Ventricular Arrhythmia. Multicenter Automatic Defibrillator Implantation Trial Investigators." *The New England Journal of Medicine* 335, no. 26 (1996): 1933–40. https://www.nejm.org/ doi/10.1056/NEJM199612263352601.

Mozaffarian, Dariush, Emelia J. Benjamin, Alan S. Go, Donna K. Arnett, Michael J. Blaha, Mary Cushman, Sarah de Ferranti, et al., "Heart Disease and Stroke Statistics—2015 Update: A Report from the American Heart Association." *Circulation* 131, no. 4 (2015): e29–322. https://www.ahajournals.org/doi/full/10.1161/cir.0000000000000152.

Mudrick, Daniel W., Bimal R. Shah, Lisa A. McCoy, Barbara L. Lytle, Fredrick A. Masoudi, Jerome J. Federspiel, Patricia A. Cowper, Cynthia Green, and Pamela S. Douglas. "Patterns of Stress Testing and Diagnostic Catheterization after Coronary Stenting in 250 350 Medicare Beneficiaries." *Circulation and Cardiovascular Imaging* 6, no. 1 (2013): 11–19. https://www.ahajournals.org/doi/full/10.1161/CIRCIMAGING.112.974121.

Mudrick, Daniel W., Patricia A. Cowper, Bimal R. Shah, Manesh R. Patel, Neil C. Jensen, Matthew J. Drawz, Eric D. Peterson, and Pamela S. Douglas. "Downstream Procedures and Outcomes after Stress Testing for Suspected Coronary Artery Disease in the United States." *American Heart Journal* 163, no 3. (2012): 454–61. https://www.ncbi.nlm.nih.gov/pmc/articles/PMC3886123/.

National Heart, Lung, and Blood Institute. "Pacemakers." Health Topics. National Institute of Health (website). https://www.nhlbi.nih.gov/health-topics/pacemakers. Accessed August 25, 2018.

Navarro, Victor J., Huiman X. Barnhart, Herbert L. Bonkovsky, Timothy J. Davern, Robert J. Fontana, Lafaine M. Grant, K. Rajender Reddy, et al. "Liver Injury from Herbals and Dietary Supplements in the U.S. Drug-Induced Liver Injury Network." *Hepatology* 60, no. 4 (2014): 1399–408. https://doi.org/10.1002/hep.27317.

Neuman, Mark D., Jennifer N. Goldstein, Michael A. Cirullo, and J. Sanford Schwartz. "Durability of Class I American College of Cardiology/American Heart Association Clinical Practice Guideline Recommendations." *JAMA* 311, no. 20 (2014): 2092–100. https://jamanetwork.com/journals/jama/fullarticle/1874510.

The New England Journal of Medicine. "Complications of Permanent Cardiac Pacemakers." Letter to the editor, 313, no.17 (1985): 1085–88.

Newmaster, Steven G., Meghan Grguric, Dhivya Shanmughanandhan, Sathishkumar Ramalingam, and Subramanyam Ragupathy. "DNA Barcoding Detects Contamination and Substitution in North American Herbal Products." *BMC Medicine* 11, no. 1 (2013): 222. https://doi.org/10.1186/1741-7015-11-222.

The NNT Group. "Coronary Artery Bypass Graft Surgery (Heart Bypass) for Preventing Death Over Ten Years." Last updated July 20, 2014. http://www.thennt.com/nnt/coronary-heart-bypass-surgery-for-prevention-of-death/.

———. "Stents for Stable Coronary Artery Disease." Updated January 8, 2018. http://www.thennt.com/nnt/stents-stable-coronary-artery-disease/.

Noheria, Amit, Peter Shrader, Jonathan P. Piccini, Gregg C. Fonarow, Peter Russell Kowey, Kenneth W. Mahaffey, Gerald V. Naccarelli, Peter A. Noseworthy, James A. Reiffel, Benjamin A. Steinberg, Laine E. Thomas, Eric D. Peterson, and Bernard J. Gersh. "Rhythm Control versus Rate Control and Clinical Outcomes in Patients with Atrial Fibrillation: Results from the ORBIT-AF Registry." *JACC: Clinical Electrophysiology* 2, no. 2 (2016): 221–29. https://doi.org/10.1016/j.jacep.2015.11.001.

Oliver, Myrna. "Robert Bruce, 87; Researcher Developed Treadmill Stress Test." *LA Times*, February 16, 2004. http://articles.latimes.com/2004/feb/16/local/me -bruce16.

OMICS International. "Atrial Fibrillation." Conferences. https://www.omicsonline .org/conferences-list/atrial-fibrillation. Accessed August 25, 2018.

Oppenheimer, Bernard S., and Marcus A. Rothschild. "Electrocardiographic Changes Associated with Myocardial Involvement with Special Reference to Prognosis." *JAMA* 69, no. 6 (1917): 429–31.

Packer, Douglas L., Daniel B. Mark, Richard A. Robb, Kristi H. Monahan, Tristram D. Bahnson, Kathleen Moretz, Jeanne E. Poole, Alice M. Mascette, Yves D. Rosenberg, Neal O. Jeffries, Hussein R. Al-Khalidi and Kerry L. Lee. "Catheter Ablation versus Antiarrhythmic Drug Therapy for Atrial Fibrillation (CABANA) Trial: Study Rationale and Design." *American Heart Journal* 199 (2018): 192–99. https://doi .org/10.1016/j.ahj.2018.02.015.

Pardee, Harold E. B. "An Electrocardiographic Sign of Coronary Artery Obstruction." *Archives of Internal Medicine* 26, no. 2 (1920): 244–57.

Parsonnet, Victor, and Jerzy O. Giedwoyn. "Pacemaker Failure Following External Defibrillation" and author reply. *Circulation* 45, no. 5 (1972): 1144–45. https:// www.ahajournals.org/doi/pdf/10.1161/01.CIR.45.5.1144-a.

Patel, Manesh R., Eric D. Peterson, David Dai, Matthew Brennan, Rita F. Redberg, Vernon Anderson, Ralph G. Brindis, and Pamela S. Douglas. "Low Diagnostic Yield of Elective Coronary Angiography." *The New England Journal of Medicine* 362, no. 10 (2010): 886–95. https://www.nejm.org/doi/full/10.1056/NEJMoa0907272.

Pollack, Andrew. "California Patients Talk of Needless Heart Surgery." *New York Times*, November 4, 2002. https://www.nytimes.com/2002/11/04/business/california -patients-talk-of-needless-heart-surgery.html.

Polyzos, Konstantinos A., Athanasios A. Konstantelias, and Matthew E. Falgas. "Risk Factors for Cardiac Implantable Electronic Device Infection: A Systematic Review and Meta-Analysis." *EP Europace* 17, no. 5 (2015): 767–77. https://doi .org/10.1093/europace/euv053.

Poole, Jeanne E., George W. Johnson, Anne S. Hellkamp, Jill Anderson, David J. Callans, Merritt H. Raitt, Ramakota K. Reddy, et al. "Prognostic Importance of Defibrillator Shocks in Patients with Heart Failure." *The New England Journal of Medicine* 359, no. 10 (2008): 1009–17. https://www.nejm.org/doi/full/10.1056/ NEJMoa071098.

Pope Alexander. *An Essay on Criticism*. London: Printed for W. Lewis in Russel Street, Covent Garden; and Sold by W. Taylor at the Ship in Pater-Noster Row, T. Osborn Near the Walks, and J. Graves in St. James Street, 1711.

Rabin, Roni Caryn. "Can You Miss the Signs of Heart Disease or a Heart Attack?" *New York Times*, April 20, 2018. https://www.nytimes.com/2018/04/20/well/live/ signs-symptoms-heart-disease-heart-attack.html.

Radder, Joseph. "Wilson Greatbatch: Man of the Millennium." *Living Prime Time*. December 1999. http://www.livingprimetime.com/AllCovers/dec1999/workdec1999/ wilson_greatbatch_man_of_the_mil.htm.

Ranasinghe, Isuru, Craig S. Parzynski, James V. Freeman, Rachel P. Dreyer, Joseph S. Ross, Joseph G. Akar, Harlan M. Krumholz, and Jeptha P Curtis. "Long-Term Risk for Device-Related Complications and Reoperations after Implantable Cardioverter-Defibrillator Implantation: An Observational Cohort Study." *Annals of Internal Medicine* 165, no. 1 (2016): 20–29.

Redberg, Rita F. "Talking about Patient Preferences." *JAMA Internal Medicine* 174, no. 3 (2014): 321. https://jamanetwork.com/journals/jamainternalmedicine/full article/1809975.

Reed, Sarah Jane, and Steve Pearson. "Choosing Wisely® Recommendation Analysis: Prioritizing Opportunities for Reducing Inappropriate Care." Institute for Clinical and Economic Review. [May 2015]. http://www.choosingwisely.org/wp-content/ uploads/2015/05/ICER_Preoperative-Stress-Testing.pdf.

Rosenthal, Elisabeth. *An American Sickness: How Healthcare Became Big Business and How You Can Take It Back.* New York: Penguin Press, 2017.

Rothberg, Michael B., Laura Scherer, Mohammad Amin Kashef, Megan Coylewright, Henry H. Ting, Bo Hu, and Brian J. Zikmund-Fisher. "The Effect of Information Presentation on Beliefs about the Benefits of Elective Percutaneous Coronary Intervention." *JAMA Internal Medicine* 174, no. 10 (2014): 1623–29. https://jama network.com/journals/jamainternalmedicine/fullarticle/1898876.

Rothberg, Michael B., Senthil K. Sivalingam, Javed Ashraf, Paul Visintainer, John Joelson, Reva Kleppel, Neelima Vallurupalli, and Marc J. Schweiger. "Patients' and Cardiologists' Perceptions of the Benefits of Percutaneous Coronary Intervention for Stable Coronary Disease." *Annals of Internal Medicine* 153, no. 5 (2010): 307–13.

Ryan, Thomas J. "The Coronary Angiogram and Its Seminal Contributions to Cardiovascular Medicine Over Five Decades." *Circulation* 106, no. 6 (2002): 752–56. https://www.ahajournals.org/doi/full/10.1161/01.CIR.0000024109.12658.D4.

Sabalow, Ryan. "Moon Loses License." (*Redding, California*) *Record Searchlight*, November 14, 2007. http://archive.redding.com/news/moon-loses-license-ep -378302418-356395691.html/.

Saint-Exupéry, Antoine de. *Le Petit Prince.* [Paris]: Gallimard, 1943.

———. *The Little Prince.* Translated by Katherine Woods. [New York]: Reynal and Hitchcock, 1943.

Scheinman, Melvin [M.], and John D. Rutherford. "The Development of Cardiac Arrhythmia Ablation: A Conversation with Melvin A. Scheinman, MD." *Circulation* 135, no. 13 (2017): 1191–93. https://doi.org/10.1161/CIRCULATION AHA.117.027956.

Scheinman, Melvin M., Fred Morady, David S. Hess, and Rolando Gonzalez. "Catheter-Induced Ablation of the Atrioventricular Junction to Control Refractory Supraventricular Arrhythmias." *JAMA* 248, no. 7 (1982): 851–55.

Schilling, Richard J., and Razeen Gopal. "Mortality and Catheter Ablation of Atrial Fibrillation." *British Journal of Cardiology* 17 (2010): 161–62. https://bjcardio .co.uk/2010/07/mortality-and-catheter-ablation-of-atrial-fibrillation/.

Schweitzer, Albert. *Kulturphilosophie.* Bern: P. Haupt, 1923.

———. *Philosophy of Civilisation.* Translated by C. T. Campion. London: Black, 1932.

Sears, Samuel F., Jessica D. Hauf, Kari Kirian, Garrett Hazelton, and Jamie B. Conti. "Posttraumatic Stress and the Implantable Cardioverter-Defibrillator Patient: What the Electrophysiologist Needs to Know." *Circulation: Arrhythmia and Electrophysiology* 4, no. 2 (2011): 242–50. https://doi.org/10.1161/CIRCEP.110.957670.

Sems, S. Andrew, Erik C. Summers, and Traci L. Jurrens. "Cardiac Stress Testing Has Limited Value Prior to Hip Fracture Surgery." Paper #49, presented at the 23rd Annual Meeting of the Orthopaedic Trauma Association, Boston, October 18–20, 2007.

Shah, Bimal Ramesh, Lisa A. McCoy, Jerome J. Federspiel, Daniel W. Mudrick, Patricia A. Cowper, Frederick A. Masoudi, Barbara L. Lytle, Cynthia L. Green, and Pamela Sylvia Douglas. "Use of Stress Testing and Diagnostic Catheterization after Coronary Stenting: Association of Site-Level Patterns with Patient Characteristics and Outcomes in 247,052 Medicare Beneficiaries." *Journal of the American College of Cardiology* 62, no. 5 (2013): 439–46. http://www.onlinejacc.org/content/62/5/439.

Shah, Bimal Ramesh, Patricia A. Cowper, Sean M. O'Brien, Neil C. Jensen, Matthew Drawz, Manesh R. Patel, Pamela Sylvia Douglas, and Eric D. Peterson. "Patterns of Cardiac Stress Testing after Revascularization in Community Practice." *Journal of the American College of Cardiology* 56, no. 16 (2010): 1328–34. http://www.onlinejacc .org/content/56/16/1328.

Shanafelt, Tait D. "Enhancing Meaning in Work: A Prescription for Preventing Physician Burnout and Promoting Patient-Centered Care." *JAMA* 302, no. 12 (2009): 1338–40.

Shaneyfelt, Terrence M., and Robert M. Centor. "Reassessment of Clinical Practice Guidelines: Go Gently into That Good Night." *JAMA* 301, no.8 (2009): 868–69.

Shannon, Maggie Oman, ed. *Prayers for Healing: 365 Blessings, Poems, and Meditations from around the World.* Introduction by the Dalai Lama. Berkeley: Conari Press, 2000.

Sheffield, Kristin M., Patricia S. Stone, Jaime Benarroch-Gampel, James S. Goodwin, Casey A. Boyd, Dong Zhang, and Taylor S. Riall. "Overuse of Preoperative Cardiac Stress Testing in Medicare Patients Undergoing Elective Noncardiac Surgery." *Annals of Surgery* 257, no.1 (2013): 73–80. https://www.ncbi.nlm.nih.gov/pmc/articles/ PMC3521863/pdf/nihms409211.pdf.

Sinclair, Upton. *I, Candidate for Governor: And How I Got Licked.* Pasadena, CA: Author, 1935.

Smith, F. M. "The Ligation of the Coronary Arteries with Electrocardiographic Study." *Archives of Internal Medicine* 22, no. 1 (1918): 8–27.

Smith, Jacquelyn. "The Best- And Worst-Paying Jobs for Doctors." *Forbes.* July 20, 2012. https://www.forbes.com/sites/jacquelynsmith/2012/07/20/the-best-and -worst-paying-jobs-for-doctors-2/#1c557431a2a3.

Sohail, Muhammad Rizwan, Daniel Zachary Uslan, Akbar H. Khan, Paul A. Friedman, David L. Hayes, Walter R. Wilson, James M. Steckelberg, Sarah M. Jenkins, and Larry M. Baddour. "Infective Endocarditis Complicating Permanent Pacemaker and Implantable Cardioverter-Defibrillator Infection." *Mayo Clinic Proceedings* 83, no. 1 (2008): 46–53.

Stergiopoulos, Kathleen, and David L. Brown. "Initial Coronary Stent Implantation with Medical Therapy vs Medical Therapy Alone for Stable Coronary Artery Disease: Meta-Analysis of Randomized Controlled Trials." *Archives of Internal Medicine* 172, no. 4 (2012): 312–29. https://jamanetwork.com/journals/jamainternalmedicine/fullarticle/1108733.

Stevenson, Lynne Warner, and Akshay S. Desai. "Selecting Patients for Discussion of the ICD as Primary Prevention for Sudden Death in Heart Failure." *Journal of Cardiac Failure* 12, no. 6 (2006): 407–12.

Stewart, Simon, Carole L. Hart, David J. Hole, and John J. V. McMurray. "Population Prevalence, Incidence, and Predictors of Atrial Fibrillation in the Renfrew/Paisley Study." *Heart* 86, no. 5 (2001): 516–21. http://dx.doi.org/10.1136/heart.86.5.516.

Stukel, Therese A., Lee F. Lucas, and David E. Wennberg. "Long-Term Outcomes of Regional Variations in Intensity of Invasive vs Medical Management of Medicare Patients with Acute Myocardial Infarction." *JAMA* 293, no. 11 (2005): 1329–37. https://jamanetwork.com/journals/jama/fullarticle/200542.

Suga, Chikashi, David L. Hayes, Linda K. Hyberger, and Margaret A. Lloyd. "Is There an Adverse Outcome from Abandoned Pacing Leads?" *Journal of Interventional Cardiac Electrophysiology* 4, no. 3 (2000): 493–99.

Tachjian, Ara, Viqar Maria, and Arshad Jahangir. "Use of Herbal Products and Potential Interactions in Patients with Cardiovascular Diseases." *Journal of the American College of Cardiology* 55, no. 6 (2010): 515–25. https://www.ncbi.nlm.nih.gov/pmc/articles/PMC2831618/.

Tavakol, Morteza, Salman Ashraf, and Sorin J. Brener. "Risks and Complications of Coronary Angiography: A Comprehensive Review." *Global Journal of Health Science* 4, no.1 (2012): 65–93. https://www.ncbi.nlm.nih.gov/pmc/articles/PMC4777042/.

Thomas, Michael P., Craig S. Parzynski, Jeptha P. Curtis, Milan Seth, Brahmajee K. Nallamothu, Paul S. Chan, John A. Spertus, Manesh R. Patel, Steven M. Bradley, and Hitinder S. Gurm. "Percutaneous Coronary Intervention Utilization and Appropriateness across the United States." *PLOS One* 10, no. 9 (2015): e0138251. https://doi.org/10.1371/journal.pone.0138251.

Tricoci, Pierluigi, Joseph M. Allen, Judith M. Kramer, Robert M. Califf, and Sidney C. Smith. "Scientific Evidence Underlying the ACC/AHA Clinical Practice Guidelines." *JAMA* 301, no. 8 (2009): 831–41. https://jamanetwork.com/journals/jama/fullarticle/183453.

Tu, Jack V., Chris L. Pashos, C. David Naylor, Erluo Chen, Sharon-Lise Normand, Joseph P. Newhouse, and Barbara J. McNeil. "Use of Cardiac Procedures and Outcomes in Elderly Patients with Myocardial Infarction in the United States and Canada." *The New England Journal of Medicine* 336, no. 21 (1997): 1500–1505. https://www.nejm.org/doi/full/10.1056/NEJM199705223362106.

Udo, Erik O., N. M. Hemel Van, N. P. A Zuithoff, P. A. Doevendans, and K. A. Moons, on behalf of FOLLOWPACE study. "Survival and Determinants of Survival in Bradycardia Pacemaker Recipients: A Nationwide Cohort Study." *European Heart Journal*, 34 no.1, (2013): 2617.

US Attorney's Office, Eastern District of Kentucky. "London Cardiologist Convicted of Health Care Fraud for Medically Unnecessary Pacemakers." US Department of Justice (website). April 16, 2018. https://www.justice.gov/usao-edky/pr/london-cardiologist-convicted-health-care-fraud-medically-unnecessary-pacemakers.

US Department of Justice Office of Public Affairs. "Medical Device Manufacturer Guidant Sentenced for Failure to Report Defibrillator Safety Problems to FDA: Boston Scientific Subsidiary Sentenced to Pay Criminal Penalty of More than $296 Million and Three Years Probation." Justice News. US Department of Justice (website). Updated September 15, 2014. https://www.justice.gov/opa/pr/medical-device-manufacturer-guidant-sentenced-failure-report-defibrillator-safety-problems.

————. "Nearly 500 Hospitals Pay United States More than $250 Million to Resolve False Claims Act Allegations Related to Implantation of Cardiac Devices." Justice News. US Department of Justice (website). Updated April 28, 2017. https://www.justice.gov/opa/pr/nearly-500-hospitals-pay-united-states-more-250-million-resolve-false-claims-act-allegations.

US Food and Drug Administration. "Development and Approval Process (Drugs)." Last updated June 13, 2018. https://www.fda.gov/drugs/developmentapprovalprocess/default.htm.

————. "FDA 101: Dietary Supplements." Last updated November 6, 2017. https://www.fda.gov/ForConsumers/ConsumerUpdates/ucm050803.htm.

van Bokhoven, Marloes A., Marjolein C. H. Pleunis-van Empel, Hèlen Koch, Richard P. T. M. Grol, Geert-Jan Dinant, and Trudy van der Weijden. "Why Do Patients Want to Have Their Blood Tested? A Qualitative Study of Patient Expectations in General Practice." *BMC Family Practice* 7 (2006): 75–75. https://doi.org/10.1186/1471-2296-7-75.

Van Gelder, Isabelle C., Vincent E. Hagens, Hans A. Bosker, J. Herre Kingma, Otto Kamp, Tsjerk Kingma, Salah A. Said, Julius I. Darmanata, Alphons J. M. Timmermans, Jan G. P. Tijssen, and Harry J. G. M. Crijns, for the Rate Control versus Electrical Cardioversion for Persistent Atrial Fibrillation Study Group. "A Comparison of Rate Control and Rhythm Control in Patients with Recurrent Persistent Atrial Fibrillation." *The New England Journal of Medicine* 347, no. 23 (2002): 1834–40. https://www.nejm.org/doi/full/10.1056/NEJMoa021375.

van Rees, Johannes B., Carel Jan Willem Borleffs, Mihály K. de Bie, Theo Stijnen, Lieselot van Erven, Jeroen J. Bax, and Martin Jan Schalij. "Inappropriate Implantable Cardioverter-Defibrillator Shocks: Incidence, Predictors, and Impact on Mortality." *Journal of the American College of Cardiology* 57, no. 5 (2011): 556–62. https://doi.org/10.1016/j.jacc.2010.06.059.

Verrilli, Diana, and H. Gilbert Welch. "The Impact of Diagnostic Testing on Therapeutic Interventions." *JAMA* 275, no.15 (1996): 1189–91.

Voet, J. G., Yves Vandekerckhove, Luc Muyldermans, Luc H. Missault, and L. J. Matthys. "Pacemaker Lead Infection: Report of Three Cases and Review of the Literature." *Heart* 81, no. 1 (1999): 88–91. http://dx.doi.org/10.1136/hrt.81.1.88.

Waldman, Peter, David Armstrong, and Sydney P. Freedberg. "Deaths Linked to Cardiac Stents Rise as Overuse Seen." *Bloomberg News*, September 25, 2013. https://

www.bloomberg.com/news/articles/2013-09-26/deaths-linked-to-cardiac-stents
-rise-as-overuse-seen.

Walters, Joanna. "Doctor Who Ordered Unnecessary Heart Surgery and Risky Tests
Jailed for 20 Years." *The Guardian*, December 22 2015. https://www.theguardian
.com/us-news/2015/dec/22/doctor-who-ordered-unnecessary-heart-surgery-and
-risky-tests-jailed-for-20-years.

Wattigney, Wendy A., George A. Mensah, and Janet B. Croft. "Increased Atrial Fibrillation Mortality: United States, 1980–1998." *American Journal of Epidemiology* 155,
no. 9 (2002): 819–26. https://doi.org/10.1093/aje/155.9.819.

Welch, H. Gilbert. "If You Feel O.K., Maybe You Are O.K." *New York Times*, February
27, 2012. https://www.nytimes.com/2012/02/28/opinion/overdiagnosis-as-a-flaw
-in-health-care.html.

Wellens, Hein J. J. "Cardiac Arrhythmias: The Quest for a Cure; A Historical Perspective." *Journal of the American College of Cardiology* 44, no. 6 (2004): 1155–63.
https://doi.org/10.1016/j.jacc.2004.05.080.

Wennberg, David E., Merle A. Kellett, John D. Dickens Jr., David J. Malenka, Leonard Mark Keilson, and Robert B. Keller. "The Association between Local Diagnostic
Testing Intensity and Invasive Cardiac Procedures." *JAMA* 275, no. 15 (1996):
1161–64.

Wikipedia. S.v. "Michel Mirowski: Medical Training." Last updated December 18,
2018. https://en.wikipedia.org/wiki/Michel_Mirowski#Medical_training.

———. "Robert A. Bruce." Last modified January 17, 2018. https://en.wikipedia
.org/w/index.php?title=Robert_A._Bruce&oldid=82085890.

———. S.v. "Siege of Leningrad." Last edited January 28, 2019. https://en.wikipedia
.org/wiki/Siege_of_Leningrad.

———. S.v. "Treadmill: Treadmills for Punishment." Last updated January 10, 2019.
https://en.wikipedia.org/wiki/Treadmill#Treadmills_for_punishment.

Wilson, Chad T., Elliott S. Fisher, Gilbert Welch, Andrea E. Siewers, and F. Lee Lucas.
"U.S. Trends in CABG Hospital Volume: The Effect of Adding Cardiac Surgery
Programs." *Health Affairs* 26, no. 1 (2007): 162–68. https://doi.org/10.1377/
hlthaff.26.1.162.

Wolf, Philip A., Thomas R. Dawber, H. Emerson Thomas, and William B. Kannel.
"Epidemiologic Assessment of Chronic Atrial Fibrillation and Risk of Stroke: The
Framingham Study." *Neurology* 28, no. 10 (1978): 973–77.

Wolferth, Charles C. "The Diagnosis and Treatment of Acute Coronary Occlusion."
Medical Clinics of North America 21, no. 4 (1937): 991–1001.

Wolters Kluwer. "Stable Ischemic Heart Disease: Indications for Revascularization."
UpToDate (website). Last updated February 18, 2019. https://www.uptodate.com/
contents/stable-ischemic-heart-disease-indications-for-revascularization.

———. "Stable Ischemic Heart Disease: Overview of Care." *UpToDate* (website). Last
updated February 18, 2019. https://www.uptodate.com/contents/stable-ischemic
-heart-disease-overview-of-care.

Wood, Francis C., and Charles C. Wolferth. "Angina Pectoris: The Clinical and
Electrocardiographic Phenomena of the Attack and Their Comparison with the

Effects of Experimental Coronary Occlusion." *Archives of Internal Medicine* 47, no. 3 (1931): 339–65.

Wyse, D. George, Albert L. Waldo, John P. DiMarco, Michael J. Domanski, Yelena Rosenberg, Eleanor B. Schron, Joyce C. Kellen, Harry L. Greene, Mary C. Mickel, J. E. Dalquist, and Scott D. Corley. "A Comparison of Rate Control and Rhythm Control in Patients with Atrial Fibrillation." *The New England Journal of Medicine* 347, no. 23 (2002): 1825–33. https://www.nejm.org/doi/full/10.1056/NEJM oa021328.

Youngson, Robin A. J. *Time to Care: How to Love Your Patients and Your Job*. Seattle: CreateSpace, 2012.

Yusuf, Salim, Deborah R. Zucker, Eugene R. Passamani, Peter Peduzzi, Timothy Takaro, Lloyd D. Fisher, Jamie L. W. Kennedy, et al. "Effect of Coronary Artery Bypass Graft Surgery on Survival: Overview of 10-Year Results from Randomised Trials by the Coronary Artery Bypass Graft Surgery Trialists Collaboration." *The Lancet* 344, no. 8922 (1994): 563–70.

Zalewska-Adamiec, Małgorzata, Hanna Bachórzewska-Gajewska, Paweł Kralisz, Konrad Nowak, Tomasz Hirnle, and Sławomir Dobrzycki. "Prognosis in Patients with Left Main Coronary Artery Disease Managed Surgically, Percutaneously or Medically: A Long-Term Follow-Up." *Kardiologia Polska* 71, no.8 (2013): 787–95. https://ojs.kardiologiapolska.pl/kp/article/view/KP.2013.0189/7409.

Zipes, Douglas P., A. John Camm, Martin Borggrefe, Alfred E. Buxton, Bernard Chaitman, Martin Fromer, Gabriel Gregoratos, et al. "ACC/AHA/ESC 2006 Guidelines for Management of Patients with Ventricular Arrhythmias and the Prevention of Sudden Cardiac Death—Executive Summary: A Report of the American College of Cardiology/American Heart Association Task Force and the European Society of Cardiology Committee for Practice Guidelines (Writing Committee to Develop Guidelines for Management of Patients with Ventricular Arrhythmias and the Prevention of Sudden Cardiac Death)." *European Heart Journal* 114, no. 10 (2006): 1088–132. https://www.ahajournals.org/doi/pdf/10.1161/CIRCULATION AHA.106.178104.

Zoll, Paul M., Arthur J. Linenthal, William Gibson, Milton H. Paul, Leona R. Norman. "Termination of Ventricular Fibrillation in Man by Externally Applied Electric Countershock." *The New England Journal of Medicine* 254, no. 16 (1956): 727–32.

Index

About the Author

J Shah is a board-certified cardiologist and a trained Epidemiologist. He was trained at Harvard Medical School and has practiced in various countries and diverse settings over the past 20 years. He is passionate about patient experience of healthcare and hopes to bring human elements back to medicine. When he is not seeing patients, he is writing, traveling or hiking. He lives in Boulder, Colorado.